AN OUTSTANDING FRAUD-The problem with

Psychiatry

Contents:

A compendium of academic papers and articles on the nature, efficacy and justification of psychiatry looking at the drug culture it encourages, the hypothesis that underline and support it, and its autocratic behaviour fixed within historical if unproven claims to scientific, empirical evidence, its connection to the state and construction and implementation of its own laws, ethical codes and rules of behaviour.

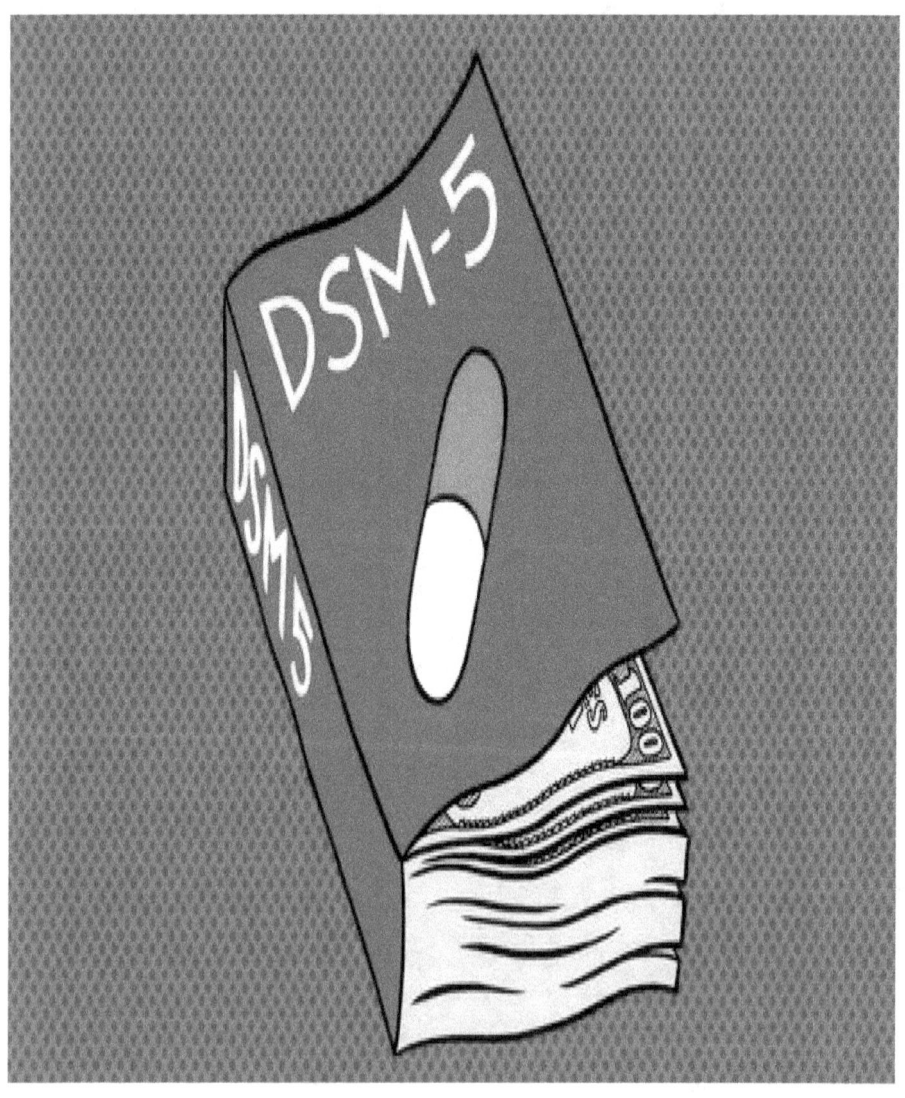

DSM-Diagnostic and Statistical Manual of Mental Disorders.

Dangers of psychotropic drugs.

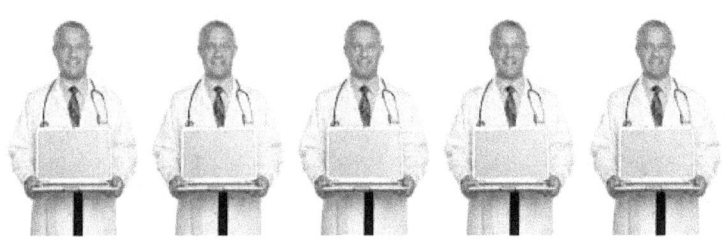

Image and branding: The medical Profession

This paper will initially review medical sites that relay official views on mental health and, while discussing their pronouncements, consider independent arguments that at times contradict official medical views. It will be seen that such sites perhaps convey an idealised view of official health providers. This paper holds that such sites encourage over-optimistic and biased perceptions. It will consider both UK and USA sites. Statements of my clients, previously active or still active patients within the mental health services, will be consulted in order to include a more complete picture. The second part of this paper will consider new research into psychotropic drugs and finally make a comparison with information provided by the above sites.

As previously active in psychotherapy and since almost equally active in providing a listening board and being an adviser to those judged mentally ill, I have become intrigued by the difference in the views of my clients on the mental health services to that of professionals involved in providing the services. It seems from what I have heard, that the mental health services are essentially controlling and function on several planes of influence with clearly doctors at the top and patients at the bottom. Of some concern to me was that patients are not listened to and ideas on mental illness were/are assumed through observation; an unscientific method surely?

According to National Health Services internet sites, in mental health, most people work in teams of 8 to 16, but patients will first see the General Practitioner (family doctor). In fact, the GP may be their first and only port of call, although several of my clients produced evidence that contradicted this claim, informing me that letters were immediately sent out to local clinics and hospitals without their permission. The GP normally sees patients for depression, according to the site, although several years ago the common mental health complaint was anxiety. Practically the same drug is prescribed for both conditions, just the names changed. None of the sites considered the tendency of the services towards fashion-based diagnosis. Nevertheless, the number of people involved in each case will be considered in a later paper. American sites assume a more in-your-face approach to actual or potential mental health sufferers, informing readers to keep a look-out for sufferers and employ caring, intrusive strategies, seemingly broaching civil rights. Readers are informed that obesity, or weight gain and loss, is *a kind of mental illness* and a proactive approach, *Show you care, connect and share.* There is a tendency to encourage self-diagnosis and diagnose others. The understanding of mental illness is spread wide. The sites project a form of paranoia, that mental illness, like aliens, is everywhere and caring is an antidote. The language on the American sites appears significantly less scientific than on the UK sites.[1] Active verbs and words of conflict are regularly employed such as:

Struggling

Warning signs

Improving lives

The essential rhetoric is of *'community'*, *interactive activity*, movement and involvement.

On the UK sites, the information is provided in a largely epigrammatical fashion, [2]which tends to encourage trust and belief in the reader. Such writing methods convey gravity and exclude doubt. [3] Words equally encouraging trust and conviction are habitually employed:

Change

Structure

[1] https://www.mentalhealth.gov/
[2] https://www.england.nhs.uk/mental-health/
[3] file:///CProcess:/Users/Dell/Downloads/Analysis_of_psychotropic_drug_advertisin.pdf

Tackling men's mental health is the lynchpin to suicide prevention. (*A statement that immediately disallows or discourages other viewpoints.*)

Also, there are few negatives used or words that might cause the reader to experience and interiorise negativity. A sensible list of reasons for mental health that allow them to reassure, not alarm. The language is moderate. It concentrates upon normative values and lifestyles. The presentation of treatment is undramatic. The site does not mention anxiety, as it would have a few years ago as depression rather than anxiety has become the fashionable go-to form of mental illness (see above). At no point would a reader feel that any of the processes are wrong or misleading, nor is there any hint of alternative ideas to those presented. The lifestyles considered are severely limited and serious presumptions are entertained of prospective patients. By and large, the services seem idealised. Of the sites, the UK one is more professional-based, formal, uncritical and free of contradiction. Both groups emphasise the frequency of mental illness.

Branding:

The many sites of the NHS in particular function as a brand, with nothing in its many pages that is critical of the services. Nearly everyone working in the NHS apparently smiles constantly. There are few unpleasantries and everyone seems to get on. It is most evidently an idealised environment with little connection to reality. As with other sites, it presents a view of generic treatments, generic solutions and exclusively generic understanding of conditions. While the American site says mental illness is everywhere, making of it a community project, the UK site is exclusive and more concerned with processes. Doctors are portrayed as of the highest efficacy. In fact, all staff are portrayed as on top of their game, without doubt or variation in character or intelligence. Clearly there is no contradiction. Primary colours are used extensively, veering deliberately away from harsh clashing or violent colours.

In both cases, fairy tale worlds are presented to the reader, where all problems are dealt with, all problems are understood. The USA sites concern themselves with prospective sufferers as consumers of health services, while the UK sites choose the term choices, that prospective sufferers have right of choice, that is they remain autonomous. In one form or another, the patient has some control. This is not my clients' experience of the services, which they describe as autocratic and top-down. [4]

---

[4] https://www.nhs.uk/Pages/nhs-sites.aspx

Processes of assimilation:

Propaganda, advertising tropes and techniques are widely employed to present service provision of mental health, although the NHS extensively uses such methods to present information. Usually, the real world is avoided. A more realistic approach[5] can be found on newspaper websites where shortcomings and failures are regularly provided. [6]

Selling drugs to GPs:

This paper has already included a paper on the advertising of psychotropic drugs [7] (authors John Quinn, Marie Nangle, Patricia R. Casey) and how they influence doctors' prescription choices. The writers reviewed three prominent journals, *American Journal of Psychiatry, British Journal of Psychiatry*, and *Irish Journal of Psychological Medicine* between February 1988 and September 1995. 2045 advertisements were considered for a variety of psychotropic drugs. They found that metaphors used for anti-depressives included 'sunshine/cloud', 'light/darkness', and 'black/white'. Similar metaphors were used for anti-psychotics such as 'storm/calm' suggesting instability and stability. The process of the drug's ingestion was also determined by metaphors. Other journals in other European countries provided the same or similar results. The authors note that the metaphors enhance and embed the advertisements intention inculcating for commercial purposes that there is only one treatment (drugs), and that multiple causes for such illnesses and variation in individual presentation is inconsequential.

Advertising insists that mental illness is a disease and ignores completely alternative therapeutic strategies. Most NHS and American websites do the same. They also avoid information that may deny the efficacy of the drugs, such as that most people do not respond to medication. The writers suggest that metaphors within journals should be dispensed with as they may influence doctors unnecessarily. But the point remains: doctors are subjected to what amounts to skilful brainwashing using considered literary techniques, as are the general public.

Although this is a short exploration, it will be continued in other papers and points to the general conservatism of doctors and the generic unwillingness to challenge perceived opinions even when it goes against possible direct experience. The very nature of the services encourages

---

[5] https://www.theguardian.com/society/2018/mar/21/damning-report-finds-serious-failings-in-nhs-mental-health-services, https://www.theguardian.com/society/2014/oct/08/nhs-mental-health-care-readers-stories
[6] https://www.nhs.uk/NHSEngland/AboutNHSservices/mental-health-services-explained/Pages/accessing%20services.aspx
[7] Quinn, Nangle, Casey.

views of unexamined personal and group efficacy with numbers, which involves whole teams, against individual experience: considered here as teams of health workers and single patients.

Doctors:

This section deals with the unusual one track-minded approach of psychiatry and its preference for dogma over empirical evidence. The profession was recently savaged by Thomas Insel, the former NIMH Director for being old fashioned in its clinical procedures, its evidence unreliable and the DSM a barrier to genuine knowledge. [8]

Doctors are invariably higher middle-class with a high-level investment in terms of time and money in their careers.[9] Some critics hold thereby that they are not arriving at objective judgements, but the subjective ones of an elite group. As I will later demonstrate their objective methodologies are really based in subjectivity concealed through the employment of apparently scientific tools. The conclusions they make through the use of these apparently scientific tools are subjective, not empirical. [10]

Being a doctor demands particularly punishing normative behavioural-expectations. The rewards of long study and demands on behaviour are high, and thereby inculcate intellectual conservatism. In terms of authoritative behaviour (that is believing instruction by senior authority figures on accepted medical ideas of the day), given both investment and loss of reward, accepting what they are taught in university and in their junior years can be done at a conscious and unconscious level. Rebellion would incur loss of status and monetary rewards.

[8] Post by Former NIMH Director Thomas Insel: Transforming Diagnosis *By **Thomas Insel** on April 29, 2013/* https://www.nimh.nih.gov/about/directors/thomas-insel/blog/2013/transforming-diagnosis.shtml

[9] https://classism.org/psychiatry-imposition-upper-middle-class-values/
[10] Why has it taken so long for biological psychiatry to develop clinical tests and what to do about it? Kapur S, Phillips AG, Insel TR. Mol Psychiatry. 2012 Dec;17(12):1174-9. doi: 10.1038/mp.2012.105. Epub 2012 Aug 7.PMID:22869033

In fact, doctors fit many conformist archetypes within the structures of internalisation, identification and compliance. Many fit into the *obedience* type, conforming to rules and select ideas, even if that is expressed within an elite group situation-similar in nature to aristocracies (Kelman: 1958[11]). Psychiatrists, in my experience, react with anger to any challenge to their professional beliefs. Effectively, they become defensive. This does seem evidence of internalisation of elite group beliefs (Deutsch and Gerard: 1955[12]), in terms of Compliance, the rewards of their profession, and obviously Identification within a small group ethos particularly involved with ideas/beliefs. [13]Many psychiatrists fit the authoritarian personality type,[14] which contrary to expectations means they believe what they are told. They belong to a demanding profession that requires certain narrow standards of behaviour, including dress code and even deportment to enforce status and respect. In order (Compliance), to fulfil an unspoken contract to receive society's benefits as physicians must accept what they are taught and if possible not challenge it. If they are taught the efficacy of drugs they believe it, the scientific inscrutability of mental health conditions they believe it. In effect, doctors represent known social and psychological behaviours of those within certain elite groupings. Unfortunately, placing themselves above such concerns, little research is done into senior, influential members of society, members of the medical profession or not, but tends to be of people much lower down.

Once they reach higher in their career, the belief in authority, which was internalised in their youth, becomes part of the fabric of their own personalities. As they age, they become more absolutist in their ideas, more convinced by the ideas they received when young.

An additional conformity is psychiatrists and GPs uncritical reliance on notes provided by peers and experts. This of course is merely anecdotal information, is subjective and cannot have any scientific basis.

General Public

---

[11] Kelman HC. Compliance, identification, and internalization: Three processes of attitude change. Journal of Conflict Resolution. 1958;2 (1) :51-60.

[12] Deutsch, M., & Gerard, H. B. (1955). A study of normative and informational social influences upon individual judgment. *The Journal of Abnormal and Social Psychology, 51*(3), 629-636.

[13] **The Oxford Handbook of Social Influence** edited by Stephen G. Harkins, Kipling D. Williams, Jerry M. Burger

[14] The Authoritarian Personality: 1950: Theodor W. Adorno, Else Frenkel-Brunswik, Daniel J. Levinson, Nevitt Sanford: Harper & Row

The wide acceptance of medical ideas on mental illness can be viewed under Legitimate authority, our relationship to those in power and that they must know what they are doing; this is certainly what gives many the right, in the public's eyes to control others; contractual obligation, they cure us, we respect them; the term buffer comes into effect because the perceived mysterious and dangerous nature of mental illness creates panic and subservience towards those who seem to have knowledge. In mental health, the resistance of a patient to conformity simply confirms their illness.

2: Doubts on the efficacy of drugs:

At this point, this paper will consider the nature of psychotropic drugs and their specific mood or mind-altering effects. In fact, they cover a wide range, from coffee, alcohol, cocaine, to tranquillizers and anti-depressives. The medical profession tends to inform the public, often through omission, that is by avoidance of the subject, that other psychotropic drugs, such as heroin and cocaine, do not work in much the same fashion and that doctor's scientific exploration of drug effects separates beneficent psychotropic drugs from maleficent psychotropic drugs. This paper considers this kind of complete separation is unlikely in view of their shared properties. Drugs subject to criminalisation and medical drugs have similar properties and function in similar ways [15] the change in supplier, doctor and drug pusher, magically appears to change a drug's essential nature.

Also, the idea that GPs will deal with mental health problems initially without involving other professionals is vigorously contradicted by my clients who insist that it is normal practice for GPs to immediately, and often against patients' desires, inform other professionals. What happens in the GPs surgery is also dependent on the GPs knowledge of mental health, which may in fact be limited. This is against the description here that promises a particular safe and benevolent environment, an ideal of behaviour and treatments.

---

[15] The Psychoactive Effects of Psychiatric Medication: The Elephant in the Room Joanna Moncrieff M.B.B.S. , David Cohen & Sally Porter. 2013.A

What if, for example, the GP makes a poor and ill-informed diagnosis, or prescribes an inappropriate drug? What if the GP is suffering dementia, is simply stupid or insufferably arrogant? The proffered scenario makes no provision for such eventualities and therefore does not provide proper forewarning. In this scenario both GPs and the service behind them are perfect.

The medical profession dictates that psychotropic drugs are scientifically proven method of dealing with different kinds of mental illness, thereby holding to a generic nature of these illnesses, or that, whatever the circumstances of each individual the illnesses are the same. The scientific basis in effect is the disease model held obsessively by the medical profession itself. But recent research has challenged the efficacy of drugs at least, and in further papers the generic nature of these illnesses will similarly be challenged.

Moncrieff, Cohen and Taylor's paper first considers the similarities between common stimulants and medical drugs, the criminalised drugs and medical drugs, pointing out that such drugs, sharing the same or similar properties, have effects on both body and mind. Psychotropic, that is mind-altering, have the same characteristics. They then discuss a number of tests of the drugs on animals and humans in the past detailing similar results, effects on cognition and perception for example. The subjective nature connected to drug taking is not, they claim, much explored outside of normal addictive processes associated with heroin and alcohol. It is agreed that these have an effect on the character of the user, but not medical drugs it seems. Independent observers note the addictive quality of all psychotropic drugs but psychiatry denies this. The perceptual alteration is on the one hand denied by doctors, but on the other hand endorsed but only if it meets their treatment paradigms. [16] In most papers reviewed, the correctness of procedure is duly met through the physician's perceptions functioning through peer-compliance but with other apparent values attached.

---

[16] The effects of Psychotropic drugs On Developing brain (ePOD) study: methods and design. Marco. E. Bottelier, et al. BMC Psychiatry. 2014. This works takes a more sceptical view than others, but most proof relies on the accuracy of imaging and perceptions thereby arising as to normality. This requires a highly subjective approach by the physician and trust that the methods correspond to the patient's subject values of integration and well-being. A number of patients were it seems misdiagnosed.

The above paper (Moncrieff, et al) considers that psychotropic drugs do not work, certainly not as people are informed and mental health workers believe. The writers first consider the effects of other psychotropic drugs, demonstrating that such drugs have both physical and mental effects. Often drugs employed for psychiatric 'diseases' are used for recreation purposes. The authors employ the term '*psychoactive*' to reference those drugs or/and the effects of drugs that produce altered emotional and cognitive states, differing from normal un-drugged states. Unlike the imaging elsewhere employed, this is genuinely empirical. The authors detail the recreational use made of a number of psychotropic drugs employed also for medical use, listing the effects noting the subjective (emotional and cognitive) effects in those who employ them for recreational use, but which are denied apparent in those who are given the same drugs for medical use. In particular they identify amphetamines and Benzodiazepines, and mention those drugs associated with 'bad' experiences-taste and effect-or dysphoria but point out that although not used recreationally they still have psychoactive affects and like all the drugs mentioned induce physical dependency. Although this is vociferously denied by the medical profession, I take a psychotropic drug, coffee, and if I do not regularly take it I frequently fall asleep and become aggressive. Imaging will not detect the changes, nor perhaps the coffee deficit. Also, the lowering of cognition and general awareness has always been ascribed to the provision of these drugs, from the outset, thereby replicating the characteristics ascribed to psychopathology. Someone who cannot feel properly would therefore suffer perceptual change. On the other side such drugs create:

.....tricyclics are strongly sedative and also dysphoric (Dumont et al. 2005; Herrmann & McDonald 1978). SSRIs and venlafaxine appear to produce a state of lethargy and indifference, coupled with an unpleasant state of agitation, tension, and hostility in some people (Goldsmith & Moncrieff 2011). An in-depth qualitative study describes the "essential lived characteristic" of being on SSRIs as "increased distance or disconnection between takers [and] their worlds" (Teal 2009, 19). Lithium produces dysphoria, lethargy, and cognitive slowing and impairment in volunteers (Judd et al. 1977;Squireetal.1980).Anticonvulsants,todaypartofthe standard maintenance treatment of bipolar disorders, show a panoply of psychoactive effects, ranging from strong sedation and cognitive slowing to anxiety and agitation (Cavanna et al. 2010).

Such states are indeed common to many psycothropic drugs. Reiterating their known subjective properties is necessary as the medical profession as a whole is at present denying what they once readily accepted. Although in known recreational drugs such as alcohol the effects on the central nervous system are accepted, the possibility of similar long term effects of medical psychotropic drugs is not dismissed but rarely considered. That these drugs do affect cognitive abilities, memory for example and calculative capacities, as well as, in extreme cases, epileptic type fits and blackouts are matters I have picked up from my clients. The medical profession determines these as part of the disease, but not anything to do with their prescriptions.

Unfortunately, the possible personality alteration due to long term usage, which I have noticed-making psychotherapy purposeless-is immediately dismissed by members of the medical profession, even though GPs have prescribed drugs with regular abandon and still do, but not necessarily for depression. In the past Valium (now on 'dangerous' lists) and Activan have been drugs of choice. If they did the same with coffee, alcohol or heroin the country would be alarmed. Partly as the result of medical neglect rather than opposition (page 441) there is little research into the subjective effects of psychotropic drugs, unlike alcohol for example.

The authors (413) bring their analytical dismemberment onto the role of the DSM, which famously includes every known mental health condition, and those waiting invention. The DSM has been a modern driver of psychiatry and also of the spread of mental health, or, at least its diagnosis. As one of the reasons for the credibility of the DSM is the present psychiatric idea that psychiatric conditions are disease based, and the drugs' efficacy is proof of that proposition, the DSM's descriptions and categorisations must be correct. If for example the psychiatrists who compile it are categorising the personality altering effects of drugs, then the DSM is exposed as merely the tool of a pseudo-science. *As psychiatry's power and prosperity is based in its scientific credential, this exposure may never occur.*

Finally, the authors call for an individual approach to mental-health problems and not the generic one espoused by psychiatry, an approach that requires genuine communication, debate and analysis not an approach similar to looking at spots and deciding someone suffers from measles. Those spots might be something else entirely. The present generic approach reflects the needs of the mental health services not those of patients.

A different look at nerves:

Recent research may raise even more questions about the use of potent psychotropic drugs but is again unlikely to stop their use as the drugs are employed to support the status of psychiatry not to cure or alleviate patient's problems. The fact that the drugs lead to long-term use and patient dependence on mental health service providers, leading to control of their lives and person, are the actual reasons they continue to be used.

The model employed by psychiatry for their drugs genuine potency may be under attack. The idea of synapses being coated for example may remain but the processes may be wrong.

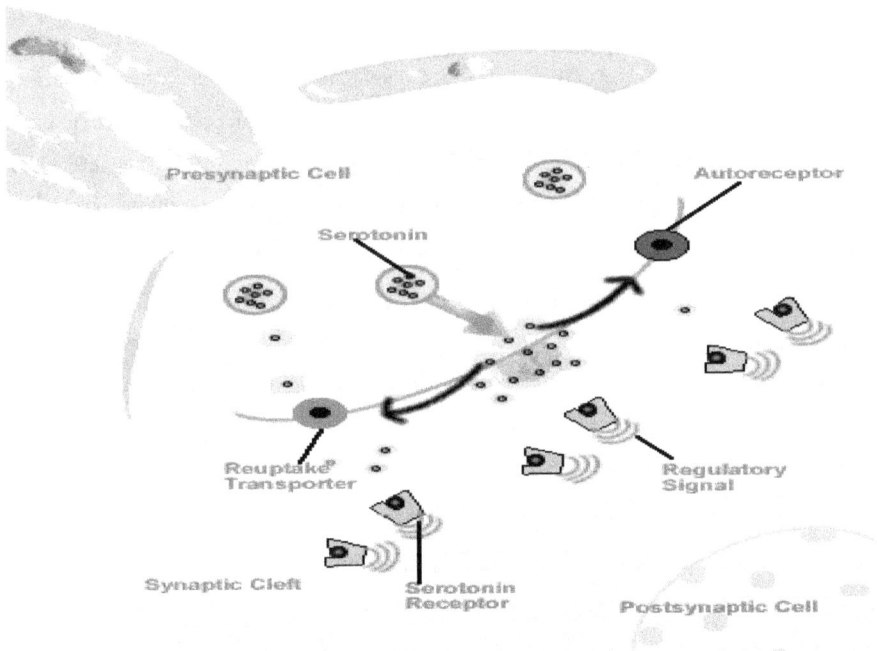

Present received model: the diagram interestingly presents a battle plan metaphor.

Psychiatry holds that neurotransmitters fire off chemical messengers, transmitting messages between neurons. They occur because of electric signals. The idea, a hypothesis then and now and not actually proven, that depression, for example, is caused by disturbances in brain circuits or neural pathways was made in the 1950s. the Serotonin hypothesis arrived in the 1960s insisting that defects in neuronal circuits using serotonin could dampen noradrenaline signalling.

Recent research denies the accuracy of this model, insisting that the transmissions are mechanical pulses not electrical signalling. If this is so, then the very basis of psychiatric beliefs may be threatened and actual effect of their drugs may be, as a growing number claim, harmful. If the signal is a mechanical impulse not an electric one, then its possible the mechanical impulse is being interfered with not the impulse. This may then cause the nerve to lessen its function, even perhaps over a long period of time go out of use. The brain thereby will be altered. The nerve signal travels down the axon's membrane but as a shock wave, squeezing the lipid molecules, changing them from fluid to liquid crystalline and causing them to emit heat. The drugs coat the transmitters and thereby affecting regulation. If in the new theory the chemicals such as serotonin are fired, that is in a mechanical process, an inhibition of that process would, it can be assumed, cause deterioration in the process itself.

Psychiatrists cannot predict what adverse side effects you might experience because not one of them knows how their drugs work. Psychotropic drugs are increasingly being exposed as chemical toxins with the power to kill. Psychiatrists claim their drugs save lives, but according to their own studies, psychotropic drugs can double the risk of suicide. And long-term use has been proven to create a lifetime of physical and mental damage, a fact ignored by psychiatrists (Moncrieff, et al).

Although dangerous toxins the drugs were introduced because they are effective from the doctor's viewpoint, not the patients. They fit the hypothesis. If they are not having a deteriorating effect on the patient's cognitive abilities then it is still possible these drugs are affecting the personality (Moncrieff, et al). If perceptions are being altered, what to? Do the drugs at least affect the patient's perception of themselves, apart from the way they are treated by doctors who commonly treat mental health patients as suffering cognitive limitations. If patients are asked about the effect of the drugs, the drugs very effects may smother cognition so any views expressed may be valueless.

DOPING THE WORLD: the monoamine hypothesis

In the 1950s it was noticed that Reserpine, a drug employed by doctors for hypertension was found to cause severe depression in 15% of patients. Now while this was not a huge number and clearly could have been explained in numerous other ways, a revolution of medical efficacy and perceptual alteration was started. [17] Reserpine is an alkaloid that was first used for hypertension but was then employed as an antipsychotic-a great leap but not one that had not occurred before. Unfortunately, although still used its use is specific as when employed extensively on pregnant women it produced or was suspected of producing brain damage in foetuses. [18]But perhaps generating a revolution is not quite that simple and a recent paper suggests that the depressgenic qualities of Reserpine was just a myth. In fact according to Alan A. Baumeister, Mike F. Hawkins and Sarah M. Uzelac[19]it was just an attempt, a successful one at that, to inculcate a *'heuristic to guide research, it enhances psychiatry's prestige, and it helps to validate and promote drug therapy for depression and other mental disorders.'* The myth was allowed to continue (the 15% is surely a giveaway) because experts at the time did not want to give up the monoamine hypothesis, which they would have had to have done, destroying modern psychiatry, millions of potential careers, in one go.

But revolutions are not produced by one event, for, about a decade afterwards, Joseph Schildkraut appeared with corroborative evidence with another drug, although years later a number of psychiatrists still suggest the evidence he produced inconclusive.[20] Dealing with this period another dissident voice appears: Shai Mulinari proffers the view that the ongoing success of the monoamine hypothesis is due to the ability *'of researchers, governmental agencies, and pharmaceutical companies to invoke theories that advance various projects and agendas.'[21]* Effectively, the monoamine hypothesis, and the other hypothesis that emanate from it are cash-cows.

[17] http://learntech.uwe.ac.uk/synapsesNeuro/Default.aspx?pageid=1925

[18] Weber-Schöndorfer, Corrina. Heart and circulatory system drugs and diuretics Drugs During Pregnancy and lactation (Second Edition) Treatment options and risk assessment.2007

[19] The Myth of Reserpine-Induced Depression: Role in the Historical Development of the Monoamine Hypothesis. Journal of the History of the Neurosciences. Basic and Clinical Perspectives. Volume 12. 2003. Issue 2.

[20] https://ajp.psychiatryonline.org/doi/abs/10.1176/ajp.122.5.509?journalCode=ajp

[21] Monoamine Theories of Depression: Historical Impact on Biomedical Research. Journal of the History of the Neurosciences. Basic and Clinical Perspectives. Volume 21. 2012. Issue 4.

Shortly after Schildkraut (1965) published his work, now known as *The Catecholamine Hypothesis* as he located catecholamine (a noradrenaline) as the relevant monoamine, the British psychiatrist Alex Coppen published a paper in the *The British Journal of Psychiatry* (1967) that emphasised serotonin (an indoleamine) as the important monoamine in psychophysiology. Combined they make up the basis of the monoamine hypothesis of depression, still rampant in psychiatry. Professional rivalry of sorts split camps in the USA and Western Europe, with the latter supporting Serotonin. The theories have been modified over time with lesions to receptors called into the argument and recently life experiences have entered the fray, bringing thereby some greater realism. Neuroplasticity, according to Mulinari (2012), is the new accepted theory, indicating a more flexible approach to the problem by psychiatrists, thereby emulating the views of their psychologist peers a hundred years after they were first mooted. Nevertheless, the chemical root remains based upon MOAIs, a monoamine oxidase inhibiter, and TCAs, tricyclic antidepressants. As yet no dominating theory of how these work has actually emerged, except that it is known that, according to Mulinari (2012), both increase catecholamine in the brain. Added to these concerns, is the growing belief that the monoamine hypothesis is simply not true, which is why it remains a hypothesis. Although many '*bad experiences*' of the drugs have constantly been recorded by patients, to the extent that its become almost a ritual (loss of emotional connectiveness for example) psychiatry as a whole has ignored such complaints and decided that, rather than being related to the drugs prescribed, the patients' sense of alienation (or panic attacks, black outs, fits-all recorded by my clients) are simply their illnesses reviving as the effects of the drugs wear out. Assessments of the nature of mental illness, the effects of drugs, consistently ignore the views of patients, but on a day to day level are based on the professional efficacy of the doctor or psychiatrist-in a method connected less to empiricism than magic. Common medical practice has been to increase drug levels. Influential voices are occasionally raised nevertheless, pointing out that there is a significant lack of conclusive proof.

Let us look at the actual evidence presented over the years, at least from Schildkraut's 1965 paper '*The Catecholamine Hypothesis of Affective Disorder: A Review of Supporting Evidence*' in which he claimed that the principal culprit for mental illness was decreased noradrenergic neurotransmission, the cure being to increase it, and in mania the culprit was elevated catecholaminergic neurotransmission. This has proved to be the abiding, classic description not just implicating two apparent opposite conditions within one remedy but then examining and explaining the biological process in the same fashion. Below is a rundown of the mechanics as understood in the present:

An action potential arrives at the axon terminal (the train travelling metaphors are important, the actions presented as those of an individual, goods or information reaching one point in their destination) the long tail coming out of the neuron down which messages are sent. This triggers the opening of calcium channels in the neurone's membrane. Instantaneously, neurotransmitters are released from storage vesicles into the synaptic cleft, the space between neurones. The neurotransmitter is diffused across the space between the neurones, binding to specific receptors on the membrane of the post-synaptic neurones. This action can result in the stimulating or inhibiting of action potential in the second neurone. (*Metaphors in these descriptions are important as they reveal mindsets-in this field the metaphors are usually connected to human movement or war/conflict*).

Two main receptors are active here, one directly linked to an ion channel in the postsynaptic membrane, while the other, not linked to an ion channel, signals the production of a second messenger. This leads to a number of changes in the postsynaptic neurone including the opening of ion channels in the plasma membrane allowing for more complex and longer lasting effects in the postsynaptic neurone.

The premise here appears to be that only two possible mechanisms operate within the human mind based it seems on a version of the pleasure/pain principle here reconstituted as Manic/Depression-the two moods the human mind seems capable of occupying. What is clear, is that the human mind has tendencies towards one or the other, it must be assumed as these are not examined, without also occupying numerous other possibilities. Disappointment for example and despair are framed within a generic Depression response, as joy, love and a sense of triumph are generically framed within an Elation, or manic response. All human emotional features can then be, and often are, classified as pathological. Moods and emotions, contrary to modern concepts, are expressed as separate-there are absolutes without co-mingling and, as will be seen, the state within the brain in which the mood message or switch emerges is the same as when it arrives. This reductionist, simplistic assessment of the human brain admits no room for the human mind.

It is the remit of the psychiatrist to say which of the above responses are framed within mania or elation, depression or disappointment. For that the physician's cultural background and experience come into play.

Before going any further, let's briefly consider the Noradrenaline hypothesis, which underlies present drug-based psychiatric medicine:

According to this theory deficiency of noradrenaline in certain brain circuits, located in the brain stem, in the *locus coeruleus*, but can travel to the limbic system (important in regulating emotions), and is connected to depression while too much produces mania. Therefore, see above, the physician has designated a demarcation line between mental health and non-health, but still refuses to define what these attributes actually consist of. They are simply free-floating responses. The more recent application to life experiences, see above, has at least removed it to some degree from the disease paradigm.

Evidence for noradrenaline depletion in depression:[22]

Levels of metabolites of noradrenaline in urine and CSF are low in depressed individuals. The condition of Depression precedes or is simultaneous with the symptoms. Both are free floating and can only be explained through a virus metaphor. So far, if perhaps the reader has noticed, there is no reference to nor evidence of an environment at this point and emotions just simply exist. Nor are emotions/moods conditioned by external conditions. This is another theory under *plasticity*.

There is greater density in specific noradrenaline receptors within the cortex of suicide victims.

Clearly, the phenomenon above probably resulted from a build-up, probably complex, of the individual´s moods and thoughts up till their final actions.

A pattern formed of 'up-regulation' (note the military metaphor) **happens whenever the neurotransmitter in synapses is extremely low, acting as a compensatory facility to pick up what is available for necessary adjustment.**

The fact that an apparently suitable mechanism exists, hardly confirms the theory's truth. Up-regulation would not then necessarily lead to depression or mania.

Drugs such as reboxetine that block this reuptake increases the noradrenaline in synapses acting as effective antidepressants in *many* people.

Therefore, only some people benefit, but which ones, well nobody really knows. Nevertheless, this is the treatment of choice-the physician's choice. The efficacy of the drug is also debatable.

Serotonin Hypothesis:

This theory also concerns itself with depletion of chemical stocks, which comes with the rationale of damaged neuronal circuits that limit noradrenaline signalling. Serotonin-producing neurones project from the raphe nuclei in the brain stem all over the brain, but, according to experts, often to brain areas to do with depression. This includes the amygdala which is connected to libido, sleep and appetite-areas of pleasure.

Clearly, this considerable scientific innovation sees human beings as entirely reactive without much clearly available cognition-a bit like very primitive organisms.

To complete this survey of received medical wisdom:

Neural Transmitters:

---

[22] Learntech.uwe.ac.uk

Neural transmitters are: Amines, Amino Acids, Peptides, and a few others.

Amines: produce Acetylcholine, synthesised choline and acetylcoenzyme A. Neurones that release acetylcholine as their neurotransmitter are normally called cholinergic neurones. These are found in the peripheral and central nervous system.

In the peripheral nervous system, acetylcholine is the neurotransmitter for:

Somatic nervous system, for skeleton muscle, pre-ganglionic nerve endings, in the parasympathetic nervous system, in the pre-post ganglionic neurones, in the central nervous system. It may be important in Alzheimer's and Parkinson's disease.

Amines produce serotonin, a monoamine. It is synthesised from tryptophan an essential amino acid in proteins. Its structure is similar to LSD. Widely found in the brainstem and cerebral cortex. It is considered to be involved in mood regulation since SSRI's (serotonin re-uptake inhibitors) are considered effective, which might be considered a circular argument. Thought to be involved in mood regulation and appetite control.

Serotonin are also, it is thought, linked to violence, and OCD.

Joanna Moncrieff, in The Myth of the Chemical Cure (2007) denies any reliable abnormalities in the serotonin system in depressed people. The limitations of genuine research into the chemical cures have been noted.

Amino Acids: involve glumate, which is an excitatory neurotransmitter, in hippocampus and cerebral cortex, but its toxicity can cause the death of nerve cells. Glycine, an inhibitory neurone found in spinal cord and brain.

GABA: synthesised from glutamate, a powerful inhibitory chemical involved in Benzodiazepines. Aspartate, similar to glutamate. Predominate excitatory neurotransmitter in spinal cord.

Glycine: smallest amino acid found mainly in inhibitory neurones in the spinal cord and brain stem. It may enable the excitatory functions of glutamate.

Peptide: Substance P-a neuropeptide with 11 amino acids

Found in synapsis within the dorsal horn of the *substantia gelatinosa*, carrying pain signals from the periphery synapses which both modulate pain and pass information. Natural opioids such as endorphins can control Substance P, decreasing release of Substance P and blocking receptors on the post-synaptic membrane.

Thyrotrophic hormone: Polypeptide. Found in hypothalamus and other brain areas. Released into the hypophyseal circulation, acting thereby on the pituitary, stimulating TSH and prolactin secretion. Aids neurotransmission into other parts of brain.

B Endorphin: Opioid peptide, formed from the molecule pro-opiomelanocortin. it is synthesised in the nerve cell body, rather than axon terminal as with the others considered here. Packaged into vesicles it is then transported along axon. Found in hypothalamus, thalamus and brain stem. Important in the modulation of pain perception and transmission. Similarities to effects of morphine.

Dynorphin: a peptide similar to B-Endorphin.

Found in similar places to B-Endorphin. It is involved in the modulation of pain.

Adenosine and Nitric Oxide may (the *may* is important) have excitatory and inhibitory effects on neurones. The Nitric Oxide is a simple molecule consisting of one nitrogen and one oxygen atom.

Adenosine contains sugars, and therefore to do with the production of sugar.

Nitric Oxide neurotransmitter for some motor neurone of the parasympathetic nervous system. In animal models, where much of this information was found, it lies in the hippocampus and contributes to long-term potentiate and learning.

Stopping signals:

The removal of neurotransmitters from synaptic gaps is achieved through diffusion, reuptake and degradation. When a neurone receives both inhibitory and excitatory neurotransmissions at the same time they join into spatial summation, temporary summation occurs when they arrive in the same pre-synaptic neurone.

Anti-depressives work by altering the number and sensitivity of post-synaptic receptors to the monoamine neurotransmitters serotonin and noradrenaline. It is considered that depressed people have hypersensitive receptors due to depleted monoamines. The level of neurotransmitters in the synaptic cleft, but work by desensitising or down-regulating the post-synaptic receptors. Prolonged lack of stimulation can produce increased cell receptors and again hypersensitivity. Inhibitory autoreceptors balance the number of neurotransmitters secreted, reducing both the synthesis and secretion of neurotransmitters.

As can be seen, the effects are within two areas, excitatory, and inhibitory, or depression. This goes along with the belief that the brain, as with all things, must be balanced to be normal. Dual systems may indeed prevail in the body but they certainly do within psychiatric thinking. Within the parameters of known mental illness, such as can be easily accepted, Manic-Depression and Schizophrenia (which themselves may not be as psychiatry claims), whereby voices (sic) can be inhibited-but not for very long from my experience, and the stabilising effects of a doctor at hand certainly helps for some sufferers. As with everything else, support systems are essential. On the surface, excitatory can seem to be an answer for Depression-if the chemicals are doing the job psychiatry claims they are. Conclusions on the effects of drugs, face to face by the doctor or through other means, does not include the numerous other factors surrounding medical and treatment events, which physicians ignore focusing on the one phenomenon-the drug. Patients thoughts and experiences are ignored, not written down or transcribed as a comment on the patient. *All is considered within the concept of the physician's magical qualities.*

The constant replenishment may indeed be due to neuronal disfunction and compensatory decrease in the number of receptors over time, but since everyone seems to require this, whatever their supposed illness, it suggests equally that it is simply a component of the drug and that bizarre behaviour that results is a consequence of the drugs not of a wearing off of their neurone-focused capacity to keep disturbed behaviour in check. Anyone, on any psychotropic drug has the same or similar experiences whether judged mentally ill or not, be it marijuana, coffee, alcohol or sex. In fact, the loss of effectiveness of the drugs may simply mean the reduction in its smothering or somatic attributes. The problems of the mentally ill simply become obvious again, after being smothered, and the consequence of retarding natural processes causes bizarre behaviour in those not judged mentally ill.

If for example the drugs have swamped traumatic memories, the individual must suddenly deal with them again, and that would prove difficult. Most of my clients exhibited bizarre behaviour while on the drugs not when off them. They also might, or probably would, need to deal with feelings again. One client told me that sex was impossible as his nerves had become far too sensitive since coming off the psychotropic drugs he had been prescribed. I was able to negotiate with clients by then novel experience of dealing with emotions, they had not experienced feelings for 10 or 20 years, by advising patience, and the brain's singular capacity to heal itself-when not prevented from doing so by drugs. The physician would have concluded the drug-induced behaviour was part of their mental illness. Unforgivably, when many GP's patients were taken off psychotropic drugs after yet another GP induced tranquilliser epidemic, most GPs washed their hands of responsibility and in general claimed withdrawal symptoms were part of their illness resurfacing.

Criticised by a number of influential voices in psychiatry, Schildkraut's ideas remain a hypothesis, [23]General Practitioners regularly prescribe the associated drugs with abandon and I have come across few GPs or psychiatrists who are even aware of the issues. They simply appear to believe what they read, which supports these hypotheses, and do not bother to investigate further. Literature from drug companies are often automatically believed with a respect for the printed word rarely found outside the Abrahamic religions. Although the consequences are regularly brushed under the carpet, the West now is one enveloping drug-culture with most of us addicted to psychotropic drugs at some point. As patients' views on these matters are generally considered of little account (one of my clients had a doctor put *rebellious patient* in their notes for refusing tranquillisers), and government and health authorities' instructions to stop are largely ignored by GPs there will be no end to the regular drug epidemics. GPs tend to be vigorous, if unthinking, supporters of the above ideas and [24]most members of the public consider this to be a proven science.

[23] https://ajp.psychiatryonline.org/doi/abs/10.1176/ajp.122.5.509?journalCode=ajp
[24] http://www.psychteacher.co.uk/abnormality/biological-treatments.html

Thomas Insel's complaints and observations (ex-head of National Institute of Mental Health (USA):

Unlike our definitions of ischemic heart disease, lymphoma, or AIDS, the DSM diagnoses are based on a consensus about clusters of clinical symptoms, not any objective laboratory measure. In the rest of medicine, this would be equivalent to creating diagnostic systems based on the nature of chest pain or the quality of fever. Indeed, symptom-based diagnosis, once common in other areas of medicine, has been largely replaced in the past half century as we have understood that symptoms alone rarely indicate the best choice of treatment.

It became immediately clear that we cannot design a system based on biomarkers or cognitive performance because we lack the data. In this sense, RDoC is a framework for collecting the data needed for a new nosology. But it is critical to realize that we cannot succeed if we use DSM categories as the "gold standard."[25]

Although Insel makes a number of pertinent points, if he appears to accept psychiatry's limited scientific data, I believe we need wholesale investigation of psychiatry and psychiatric drugs. This I believe is essential if only to break psychiatry's strange connections in public consciousness, which in the main believes that psychiatry is scientifically based when really it has little genuine scientific authenticity.

Proof:

There is here a lack of proof and most responsible commentators use words such as *'belief'* or some other qualifying word or phrase. The scientific testing has been on animals, usually with the results examined according to imaging that tends to substantiate received ideas. The first testing of Reserpine, according to Mulinari (2013), was performed on laboratory animals, inducing sedation. This was apparently seen as a form of animal depression-reeling the world into a Monty Python kind of scientific reality. This has remained common practice. By then, psychiatrists, wholly unable to back-up their supposed expertise with results, grasped at the Holy Grail placed before them! Results from here on were laboratory based, even if the laboratory was the psychiatrist's office with the psychiatrist the only determiner of illness/wellness/and the effects of treatment. In this way, psychiatrists could at last own *'reality'* and make it into whatever they desired. The pressures on doctors to accept superior's and peer beliefs are immense but also part of the invisible professional contracts a physician of any kind makes as they climb the often-demanding medical career pole, dissension can bring problems, and throughout the history of medicine *'bad medicine'* has been as eagerly accepted as *'good medicine.'*

Mulinari (2013) considers briefly the reductionist nature of the theories (shockingly successful given that they reduce human beings to light switches), acknowledged by both Schildkraut and Coppen. There were then as now a number of contradictory observations about the efficacy of their diagnosis. One problem was that the drugs were instantaneous but improvement was not, the other problem, already visited by both Moncrieff and myself, are criminalised drugs which

[25] https://www.nimh.nih.gov/about/directors/thomas-insel/blog/2013/transforming-diagnosis.shtml

appear to have the same properties. On the surface, magic is at work, for if the pusher is a doctor the drugs work miracles, if a street-corner pusher hooded and surly, then a social disaster. Cocaine blocks the uptake of norepinephrine and dopamine but apparently does not function as an antidepressant.

The negative affect of psychotropic drugs on society has been immense but complex, caught up as it is in concepts of medical trust, and the sheer complexities of modern medicine. According to Mulinari(2013), the problem was moved to one side, and effectively has been since. There were additional problems with the original research in that reserpine-induced depression in animals was caused by depletion of noradrenaline when in fact it was identified as depletion of dopamine, failing to convert into noradrenaline because the normal processes were block by the reserpine. In the early 1970s reviews were written on the effects of psychotropic drugs on depression sufferers, reflected on by Thomas Ban, a veteran psychiatrist, which indicated that only 1 out of 3 patients responded to drug treatments. By this time, drugs were fast becoming the only treatments offered, their reputation for efficacy growing until now only a few people are opposed, drowned out perhaps by too many self-serving voices. In the UK, in order to obtain any treatment people must go through their GP-there is therefore no real choice available unless someone goes private.

Prescribing drugs take little effort, produces immense revenue for an economy, and all in all little actual thinking, insight or testing is required.

To state that the reasoning is flawed (Mulinari, 2013), is also to state that by and large the evidence is actually non-existent and what there is can easily be explained in other ways. The fact that one phenomenon occurs, does not mean another does or has, especially if the second phenomenon is not a general response or when it is limited to certain laboratory conditions. Psychotropic drugs produce change, that is their nature, but it does not mean that a miracle has occurred as the changes can be symptomatic or not the changes looked for at all, fitting desired outcomes by either coincidence or in the way of someone standing near an accident-they are there, are visible but play no part in events unless identified as so doing. Proximity does not mean efficacy. In addition, if I drink loads of coffee for a week and suddenly stop my mood will shift as a consequence but that does not mean I am suddenly unwell. If I take coffee again it does not mean that my perked-up state means I am now well, or relieved of any internal angst. The angst had distinct causes. If my monoamine is depleted thereby it does not mean that that had or has anything substantial to do with either observed mood. In fact, it is not an affective state, but a physiological one mimicking an affective state.

The pain/pleasure[26] attributes of the neurones involved seems at first glance an unlikely combination for the fixed moods of pathology. These neurones are generally considered complementary, one reason for their use as recreation. They certainly will function together-eating chilli is painful and pleasurable, watching horror movies for some is painful and

---

[26] Pain, Pleasure, and Unpleasure David Bain & Michael Brady Published online: 9 February 2014 # Springer Science+Business Media Dordrecht 2014

pleasurable. The cross-overs are often unique. They point in fact to the mind's complexity, not its simplicity.

Is the messaging responding to anything viable, say a traumatic event, then clearly it is the event that causes imbalance not the neurological flaws. Any such event would be met with both pleasurable messengers as well as those of pain, there B-Endorphin would bring the necessary sense of well-being, but as their regulating properties are synchronised how precisely would they not be certainly if there is separation as psychiatry believes?

This instead is perhaps an interesting example of a powerful group (psychiatry/medical profession) controlling information and public thinking as a consequence of public trust and respect, and the desires of many groups to solve what may be unsolvable by present methods and mindsets-*what is mental illness?* It is about the restructuring of reality to inform status: careers, power and numerous *other factors that make life good for an elite group.*

Patients' experiences:

One of my clients, the victim of highly abusive parents, was given drugs by psychiatrists who according to my client seemed to make-up his symptoms and asked no pertinent questions. They judged his parents on the manner in which they presented themselves, never asking them any questions, taking the general attitude as if the boy had measles. While resident in a hospital for two months-a refuge at the time from his parents-he was subjected to drug treatment. Although little more than a child, he would have been one of the earliest victims of these drugs. When he left the hospital and of course no longer received the drugs he found himself assaulted by overwhelming crippling anxieties. He suddenly found it impossible to leave his home so profound were the bizarre feelings. Off hand, it appears he became addicted. These drug-induced symptoms were recorded as clear signs of psychosis with terrifying consequences for my client. Little more than a boy at the time, they destroyed him.

For more on these matters: *International Journal of Risk & Safety in Medicine 29 (2018) 175–180 DOI 10.3233/JRS-180018 IOS Press 175 SSRI and SNRI withdrawal symptoms reported on an internet forum.* Tom Stockmanna, Dolapo Odegbarob, Sami Timimic and Joanna Moncrieff. Many people, suffering from the effects of psychotropic medical drugs has been relabelled-usually as psychotic. The more drugs given out, the more mental illness there seems to be. Is it the effects of the drugs? *'They won't do any harm and might do some good': time to think again on the use of antidepressants? Hugh Middleton and Joanna Moncrieff. https://www.ncbi.nlm.nih.gov/pmc/articles/PMC3020050/pdf/bjgp61-047.pdf*

A number of psychotropic drug addiction epidemics have consumed millions in the UK over several decades[27], each caused by General Practitioners. This is a repeated phenomenon and, there is little doubt, has been replicated throughout the West and is now it seems appearing in the East through the extension of western medicine.

---

[27] https://www.benzo.org.uk/vot1.htm

Empirical evidence/fantasy:

In this final part I will consider a number of pertinent views on the prescribing of psychotropic drugs, their legitimacy and efficacy. In addition, I will include my own direct experiences with numerous clients over a number of years.

Psychiatry has tended to lack an overarching ideology beyond assumptions of knowing how to control, in effect managerial, madness. In the 19th century, alienists or mad doctors, the first appellations of psychiatrists, claimed authority through the management of the mad. Around them psychology and psychodynamic psychology developed gaining notice and following. It was not until the 1950s that psychiatry stepped out of the shadows as the weird old uncle, the mad doctors who ran asylums with nothing pertinent to say. In the 19th century they became infamous for locking up unwanted wives, rebellious daughters and monied relatives under the pretence of their being mad. They did not have a high reputation, but it was a dirty job and someone had to do it.

Psychotropic drugs, vigorously marketed by the drug companies, appeared and suddenly psychiatry had a believable tool instead of water-boarding, used frequently, lobotomies, ECT, and all sorts of invasive treatments which if they did not cure as likely as not killed. Psychiatry clearly felt that patients needed to suffer to become sane again. And boy, did they suffer! Drugs were comparatively civilised, even if they were habitually used by authoritarian governments to break defectors and agitators.

At first, as Joanna Moncrieff remarks, it was accepted by doctors that all the drugs did was block out disturbing thoughts and/all unsettling feelings. They were given to lonely housewives in high rises, cut off from the greater world, their lives hopeless and pointless. The majority of course became addicted to the blue pills willingly supplied by GPs. In a strange kind of support for earlier interpretations, Moncrieff, defines therapeutic drug use into the disease-centred approach and a drug centred approach, the former is what psychiatry claims to be doing and the latter is what they are actually doing.[28]   The disease-centred hypothesis is fairly recent. Psychiatry decided that there was a science behind the incessant doping regimes and at this junction, psychiatrists claimed the loftiest positions of science and of experts in human biology. Doping patients effectively controlled them and made their work easier. But the more they doped, the greater the number of the mentally ill. Numbers grew exponentially. [29]

At first psychiatrists accepted the effects of powerful psychotropic drugs as being less side effects than their main purpose, to render controllable the difficult and disturbed patients, and in many ways limit their suffering. It seemed to make everyone's lives better. It appeared a genuine solution. As the practice acquired a greater and deeper rationale, the Monoamine

---

[28] www.psychologytoday.com/us/blog/rethinking-mental-health/201602/joanna-moncrieff-the-myth-the -chemical-cure
[29] PSYCHIATRIC DRUGS AND COMMON FACTORS: AN EVALUATION OF RISKS AND BENEFITS FOR CLINICAL PRACTICE. Sparks, A. Jacqueline, Duncan, Barry. L. Cohen, David. Antonuccio, David. O. Psychiatric Drugs and Common Factors.

Hypothesis, they acquired greater prestige, bigger research grants, bigger salaries and prospects. After two centuries, they were legitimised. They moved out of the shadows and into the forefront of society.

My practice demonstrated to me that the drugs appeared not to do what psychiatrists were claiming they did. All they did was smother people: overwhelm thoughts and feelings. People's identity and potential disappeared under Valium, Ativan and an assortment of other less well known concoctions. Tranquilliser addiction became rampant.

In my practice I noted that psychiatry found it difficult to let patients go; in effect once someone was diagnosed they stayed within the parameters of the diagnosis; therefore I tended to discourage involvement with psychiatry. In fact, research has demonstrated that those that come under the generic umbrella of depression tended to recover far quicker without psychiatric help than those who received it (Sparks, el al). I saw that drugs were the main problem. Sparks et al (2000) add: ' *the common assumption of antidepressant efficacy is inconsistent with emerging observational and meta-analytic data. Kirsch and Sapirstein (1998), in a meta analytic review of 19 studies involving 2,318 people, showed that 75% of the response to antidepressants was duplicated by placebo.*' It is likely that most successes of psychiatry are due to placebo activity: often just a supportive doctor.

Another reason is possibly related to professional note-taking, a recognised procedure amongst doctors. The note-taking involves doctors or senior staff passing notes between each other bearing anecdotal information that hardly qualifies as scientific. As in the previous paper I stressed that doctors tend to fit authoritarian type personalities, that is they believe what superiors or even peers tell them, anyone they assume has authority; this is a dangerous habit as reality is continually reconstructed. Neither the patient, nor anyone associated with them can make correctives. Here, magic appears to enter the equation, although an equally conclusive metaphor is the old boys' club or network. Counter intuitively, psychiatrists tend to have no knowledge nor understanding of psychology and seem pathologically unable to perceive the harm they do to others. Too often their own perceptions are structured upon their authority, and therefore insight is constructed upon their own status. These are generic problems.

Further research (Sparks, et al) demonstrates that there is no evidence to support psychotropic drug efficacy, and this has proved to be my own observation. There is no evidence to prove any of the hypothesis itemised here (201), except anecdotal evidence from the drug companies and the medical profession as a whole-but not entirely. Such negative evidence will not affect mind-sets or procedures as psychiatry tends, fragmented into authoritarian types, to attach itself freely to dogma. Responding to status rather than evidence will construct dogmatic responses, especially when contradiction emerges.

Conclusion:

My own experience with patients and from several years of consulting material that has analysed psychiatry and the medical profession, demonstrates that the hypothesis examined here cannot be accepted. I cannot see any possible reason that pain and pleasure monoamines, complementary in the human brain, should be involved in the extremes of Depression and Manic Depression, or that medical drugs should operate so differently to criminalised and recreational ones. My observations told me they function in much the same way. It seems that the ideologies are framed around psychiatric authority and status rather than empirical fact. My wider examination of the medical profession demonstrates that the employment of psychotropic drugs, the expansion of ideas of mental illness throughout society, are inseparable from the way the medical profession as a group functions, expanding the status and influence of the group itself. Joanna Moncrieff[30] insists that her review of the disease-centred drug hypothesis, which this paper has considered, demonstrates that the idea evolved out of the vested interests of state (population control as in the 1980s during a period of extreme unemployment when some of the first tranquilliser epidemics occurred), the pharmaceutical industries pushing vested interests through government officials (Tony Blair, ex-Prime Minister), and the psychiatric system, which gave them much greater influence and respect. My extensive research indicates the correctness of Joanna Moncrieff's view that the drug therapy employed by psychiatry with its disease paradigms is closely concomitant with not simply psychiatrist's expansion of status and influence, but the state's need to stem issues concomitant with an increasing population. Evidence of scientific behaviour in much of what the medical profession does (outside of externally driven technological advances) throughout the modern era is far more difficult to find than commonly believed. Many medical ideas invariably have a self-serving impetus.

Clients who become involved with the medical profession never get better because the system demands they remain ill, while those I stop from becoming involved or can wean away from professional medicine lead happy, fulfilled lives. Part of the problem is the employment of drugs that from my experience have a corrosive, debilitating effect on the human personality. Lives become empty, fulfilling psychiatric dogma. Your psychiatrist, and mental health systems as a whole, need fodder, more than people's normal and healthy desire to become fodder. Each recruit confirms their expertise and status.

---

[30] The Myth of the Chemical Cure: A Critique of Psychiatric Drug Treatment. 2007. Palgrave.

This most uncertain of all sciences.

Introduction:

This paper explores the veracity of psychiatric ideas and practices through consideration of psychiatric ideas and thinking as expressed through three psychiatric papers addressed principally to the monoamine hypothesis. It will consider the validity of extrapolating ideas on human mental functions from research on animals, and the dangers involved.

The methods used are an examination of the scientific propositions of the three papers, chosen at random but reflecting different time periods and psychiatric thinking, an examination of alternative perspectives and textual examination of language used. Opposing views and in-depth examination of attitudes and ideas will be highlighted. The observed effects of psychotropic drugs on clients will complete this examination.

Papers considered:

These papers, asserting proof in one form or another of the Monoamine Hypothesis, have been chosen at random from past papers in the Lancet, and from academic sites, covering a period of 45 years:

Paper 1: Short Communication. Concentrations of NE and 5HT in the contused sheep spinal cord: status of the Monoamine Hypothesis. [31] Apart from the ethics of the experiments, inflicting severe injuries on sheep, cats and dogs, the conclusions seem localised and on the surface bear little genuine confirmation of the Monoamine Hypothesis. It seems an isolated experiment conducted to confirm or deny previous experiments. Its positive conclusions are difficult to accept in the circumstances.

Paper 2: A Monoamine Hypothesis for the Pathophysiology of Paraphilic Disorders. [32]

Apart from analysing a paper on paraphilia, this section considers the possible un-scientific nature of the DSM.

---

[31] Kidman, Hinwood, Yeo. Journal of Neurochemistry.1976. Vol 27. Pages 293-294. Pergamon Press. Great Britain.
[32] Kafka, Martin P. MD. Archives of Sexual Behaviour. Vol. 26. No 4. 1997.

The general hypothesis behind the as yet unidentified illness alone provides an insight into psychiatric diagnosis that is pervaded by descriptive summaries that tend to go unchallenged, replete with undocumented claims. The terms used are generic suggesting each person suffering from the specified illness acts in the exact same way as another person suffering from the illness or indeed anyone with behaviour resembling the assumed symptoms of illness. This provided example is gender based without any rationale provided other than the common prejudice that men are more sexually inclined than women towards different forms of sexual behaviour such as masturbation, and promiscuity. The writer mistakes identification by the courts of those who engage in the recognised if doubtful forms of paraphilia (a mental health designation that can be only considered appropriate in its criminal expression) and within the writers more extensive understanding of paraphilia based on the DSM. The writer takes the view that promiscuity, in line with an interest in pornography, are psychiatric illnesses that go under the heading of Paraphilic Disorder-or love of unusual sex. This is a moral position only, with variable reactions and understandings.

A medical dictionary, taking its definitions from DSM-5, describes the condition as involving not simply fantasies, but also the use of non-human objects, masochism, sadism, transvestic fetishism, frottereurism, exhibitionism, voyeurism. Within reason, all of these feelings and acts are common in most human populations. Unless taken to ludicrous extremes, none can reasonably be seen as necessarily manifestations of mental illness although some can be viewed as criminal acts. Most psychiatric definitions involve this all-inclusive nature and are thereby meaningless.[33] These matters are rarely publicly debated, unless brought into a law court to decide a case. Psychiatry comes to certain conclusions on human behaviour without any attempt at collaboration or communication devising often unsupported views on human nature. Unfortunately, this means any exhibited behaviour, if seen as exhibiting excess, can be re-constructed as mental illness. Cross dressing (transvestic fetishism) is now seen as normal, and the use of objects for sexual gratification is the accepted domain of many teenage boys. There is no concept here of the division of public and private activity found in law courts. Although frottereurism (rubbing genitalia against someone else in a bus or train for example) is disagreeable, it remains an enormous leap, although the writer has included time and internal feelings of the culprit, to classify it as a mental illness. It might be a stupid prank, a dare, or the dubious actions of an inveterate risk taker, or, if repeated, a proviso of the author, the activities of a disagreeable character.

'Paraphilias are socially deviant, repetitive, highly arousing sexual fantasies, urges, and activities that have a duration of at least 6 months. In addition, paraphilias must be accompanied by clinically significant distress or impairment in social, occupational, or other areas of interpersonal functioning (American Psychiatric Association [APA], 1994, pp. 522-532)'.[34]

---

[33] Miller-Keane Encyclopedia and Dictionary of Medicine, Nursing, and Allied Health, Seventh Edition. © 2003 by Saunders
[34] Appended to the essay's introduction.

The provision of time and other factors still does not place it within mental illness paradigms. The DSM's understanding of perversion, except for two of the models above, has not stood the test of time but are merely evidence of common prejudice. Opinion, which the DSM is full of, is not scientific. Previous dominating concepts of character provide a more satisfactory estimate of such activities.

The paper examines treatment of the above disorders with monoamine interpretations. By the 1970s monoamine interpretations of mental illness were perceived of as leading to a cure-all. The statements above are epigrammatic and deny any possible contradiction of the physician's viewpoint, assigned condition or the need for further examinations and viewpoints to be established. There is in effect no room for *falsification*. The experiments with rats rarely if ever include attempts at falsification, an accepted scientific procedure. Many aspects of the experiments are not addressed, as commonly they would be. The process tends to be: An illness has been discovered, within generic paradigms it/they look like this. In fact paraphilia could simply be itemising the known activities of easily aroused teenage boys or those who enjoy experimenting in their sex lives, but the language presents what is sometimes normal activity in an abnormal fashion. The descriptions are symptom based and insistent on free-floating processes. There is no linked narratives, reasons for categorisation or proof provided other than determinist viewpoints that demand the reader's acquiescence in the physician's judgement. That in fact is where proof lays.

It is highly possible that here as in other instances monoamine activities are secondary to other processes not identified by clinicians-constructs, concepts, intentionality, prejudices and misunderstandings.

Further; a view of the paper's introduction:

'*A monoamine pathophysiological hypothesis for paraphilias in males is based on the following data: (i) the monoamines norepinephrine, dopamine, and serotonin are involved in the appetitive dimension of male sexual behavior in laboratory animals; (ii) data gathered from studying the side effect profiles of antidepressant, psychostimulant, and neuroleptic drugs in humans suggest that alteration of central monoamine neurotransmission can have substantial effects on human sexual functioning, including sexual appetite; (iii) monoamine neurotransmitters appear to modulate dimensions of human and animal psychopathology including impulsivity, anxiety, depression, compulsivity, and pro/antisocial behavior, dimensions disturbed in many paraphiliacs; (iv) pharmacological agents that ameliorate psychiatric disorders characterized by the aforementioned characteristics, especially central serotonin enhancing drugs, can ameliorate paraphilic sexual arousal and behavior.*'

Consequent to this the reader's worst anxieties have been aroused, and by now they are imagining all kinds of behaviour that in fact may not be referenced or if referenced true. It is the language the reader is responding to and the structure of the sentences. Sexual appetite referenced repeatedly indicates the worst scenarios, repetition repeatedly used-impulsivity, anxiety, depression, compulsivity and pro (?) anti-social behaviour. The last seems to mean they are for anti-social behaviour not against it. By now, no doubt you are thinking *'Lock them up, they are clearly dangerous.'* But the reader is responding to descriptive techniques not scientific care, objectivity and scrupulousness. In fact so far we have a piece written for effect. There are language techniques galore such as rhetoric and rule of three and repetition. It is a biased narrative to, it seems, construct or support an imagined psychiatric disorder. This is not a real person, or real people, with a host of variant qualities but personified illness. Symptoms projected into an individual who may or may not exist in part if not the whole. At best this is an archetype, a half-human, half-animal driven by instinct.

This is interesting stuff. Three of the main monoamines are selected but realistically do they actually do what the writer claims? Certainly, if it does in laboratory animals it must also have the same effects on human beings, as surely we are animals too, and many of those suffering paraphilia are perhaps closer to animals than we are (sic). What reason do they have to believe that the drugs work or will work. We already know they do not work on everyone, but so far there is no sense of that here.

The range of behaviours the writer associates with this condition is extensive, and the range even more so. Criminal acts are conflated with ones normally connected to hedonism. Paedophilia is dubiously connected to sexual promiscuity, and any and all sexual activity determined by the writer as excessive is also then determined as mental illness. This does appear subjective even though referenced appropriately. There is no consensus here nor would it appear scientific justification. At the end of the first part of the essay another rule of three is employed-aggression, sadism and pornography. From my understanding, none of these constitute separately or together mental illness. Is sexual promiscuity really a mental illness, and is not the piece a prime example of a narrow concept of morality used to justify a diagnosis doubtful on all possible levels. The use of heightened negatives to convey the dangers and disturbed nature of a considerable range of sexual behaviours raises many doubts. This certainly is not science! The piece is mainly concerned with paedophilia, which perhaps should be separated from the other so-called illnesses.

Eventually, the writer gets to the main point of the text, which is the declaration that these disorders are caused by a disturbance of the central serotonin neurotransmission. What evidence is there for this? Perhaps you have already guessed-the evidence is found in animals. How? Also, the writer insists, in human males on antidepressants, psychostimulant and neurolyptic exhibit some of the *animal instincts* of paraphilia. Clients of mine have noted such changes in themselves suggesting there is a cross-over between psychotropic drugs and mental health symptoms. Consequently, the effects of psychotropic drugs can be confused with psychiatric illness. Again, notice the strange language employed by the writer, the constant conflating of human and animal behaviour within parameters of sexual excess.

The writer focuses on rats which he stresses are most like humans in their sexual behaviour. He does not explicate why he says that, but he has probably met more rats than I have. But the writer does allude to the compulsiveness of male rats' sexual behaviour with males increasingly mounting females, similar one imagines to Bonobo Chimpanzees who clearly suffer habitually from paraphilia and the wonder is that attention has not so far been directed towards this specifically anti-social animal type. Of course their activity represents interactive programming that the writer seems unaware of; the Bonobo Chimpanzee is closely related to human beings and their behaviour appears to be a variation on social interaction, one of the main attributes of human beings, this understandably cannot be appropriate. He does appear to believe human males and animals have similar sexual focus, which he interprets negatively. That extremely active sexual behaviour might not be a bad thing seems not to occur to the writer.

Perhaps promiscuity in humans serves the same purpose as in Bonobo chimps? Also, the writer, common in psychiatry, does not bother with alternative observations such as constant lighting having an effect on rat's sexual behaviour[35], none of which is then extrapolated onto human beings as a means of controlling human sexual behaviour. Nor is there any attempt by the author, again common in psychiatric papers, to consult or reference the views of acknowledged experts on human sexual behaviour. I have looked at one example at random that conceives of human behaviour as complex and driven by numerous factors.[36]

The author comes then to human beings and the application of immense research into treatment of paraphiliac sufferers. The author admits:

The neuromodulation of sexual desire in men and women is poorly understood in comparison to laboratory mammals. The elucidation of the biological mechanisms that determine human sexuality are hampered by limitations in the selectivity of biological probes, undesirable side effects of selective biological agents, as well as the absence of a noninvasive methodology to identify, localize, and selectively affect the brain areas most responsible for the substrates of sexual appetite and copulatory responses (Everitt and Bancroft, 1991). For example, there is less direct evidence that diminished central serotonin may increase sexual desire and performance in the human species (Everitt and Bancroft, 1991; Segraves, 1989). The use of PCPA in human males as a probe for sexual behavior mediated by central serotonin has produced negative results in comparison with experiments with laboratory mammals (Benkert et al, 1976; Cremata and Koe, 1966). In addition, I could not find studies that specifically measure monoaminergic metabolites or utilize biological probes to provoke monaminergic neurotransmission in male paraphiliacs. Such studies are clearly needed to support or revoke the hypothesis proposed in this manuscript. Despite these limitations, data supporting this hypothesis are presented below.

Although the writer thankfully and belatedly admits that without further corroboration the case is not proven, he fails to wonder if the very methodology might be to blame. In fact, this is usually as far as research goes in proving the monoamine hypothesis-the self-defeating acceptance that rats are not like human beings or human beings rats. The writer nevertheless informs the reader that there is abiding or at least sufficient proof that:

---

[35] Fantie, Brown, Moger. Constant lighting conditions affect sexual behaviour and hormone levels in sexual male rats. Departments of Psychology, Physiology and Biophysics, Dalhousie University Halifax, Canada. 1984 Journals of Reproduction and Fertility Ltd.

[36] Gray, Peter. Evolution and Human Sexuality. Yearbook of Physical Anthropology. 2013.

The serotonin-reuptake inhibitors, clomipramine and fluoxetine, increase postsynaptic serotonergic effects and have been reported to produce a high frequency of human sexual dysfunction side effects including the cluster of loss of sexual desire and impaired copulatory response in males (ejaculatory delay, erectile dysfunction, and anorgasmia) (Jacobsen, 1992). These reports support the observation that enhanced central serotonin neurotransmission reduces or inhibits sexual desire and associated sexual performance behaviors.

Equally there is some abiding proof that castration has the same effect but what that tells us beyond reflections on the mentality of the castrator and the induced depression into the victim I am not sure. While my words may seem flippant this is really the level, behind the proliferation of jargon, on which these experiments are pitched.

Within all this concentration on monoamine terminology is an interesting assertion that dopamine agonists such as L-Dopa when employed to treat men increases, as noted, sexual behaviour. Remember we are not dealing here with the more horrendous examples of excessive sexual behaviour but also sexual promiscuity, a relatively harmless recreational pastime between consenting adults. The main trait recognised by this paper is impulsivity, but apart from linking this to some extremes of sexual behaviour it takes a general view of it as a '*bad thing*'. Impulsivity is a sign of mental illness, not perhaps a sign of a '*fun personality*'. The writer makes no attempt to deal with the semantics or psychological and philosophical issues involved and quite rightly as he has probably not, and neither have I, ever seen a rat reading a book.

Nevertheless, so far we have learnt that some chemicals cause arousal in a variety of animals and can cause arousal (fantasies, etc,) in men. Similarly some chemicals have the reverse effect on both animals and men. Women play very little part here as the writer has decided they are not as likely to have fantasies as men, or act on them. What do women say on this?

Rebecca Plante reviews an idea here based on the theory of Adam Isiah Green's '*Bourdieusian concepts—habitus and capital—to analyze sexual worlds as arenas where "collective sexual life" occurs. This consists of "space" and interactions, real and virtual, along with "sites, networks, institutions, and subcultures within which intimate partnerships are forged"* ' which attempts to explain human sexuality in interactive environments, based of course on consent. As the writer of the piece being analysed, common to psychiatry, sees all excessive sexual behaviour as paraphiliac, thereby subject to categorisation under mental illness, all these and the author of the theory must be mentally ill. [37] The writer of the article under review has not consider widening his net to discover what others think, and compare and contrast. Psychiatry as a rule does not do that. It states a particular categorisation, as can be seen in the DSM, decides the behaviour traits consistent with that categorisation and creates yet another form of mental illness. Re. the Daily Mail on 11th September 2018, introducing in its Good Health section a new mental illness-hoarding. Well maybe, but since psychiatry's usual treatment methods are drugs, and more drugs, especially for the poor, than perhaps not.

Sex offenders:

The crux of this paper is here reached, as the main theme has been the treatment of sex offenders. As much as we may deplore their behaviour, assigning them to a framework of

[37]Sexual Fields: Toward Sociology of Collective Sexual Life. Book Review. Ed. Adam Isiah Green. Chicago, IL. University of Chicago, 2014.

mental illness is a subjective consideration and within the text the only verifiable treatment considered is chemical castration. If you are of the '*they deserve it and worse type*' you may think that is fine, but here we are discussing the appropriateness of treatments not justice and the writer is, or appears to be, unaware that is what he is concentrating on. Disapproval of actions does not mean we have to categorise those we disapprove of as suffering from mental illness of one form or another, but that is what psychiatry does. Effectively, there is more than a hint of moral judgement in the writing.

The effects of the identified monoamines has been to either increase or decrease sexual arousal, not to provide any understanding beyond the suggested role of monoamines. The writer has no interest in the human mind, nor any apparent awareness that it exists. The conflating of promiscuity with deviance is of course ridiculous.

'*There are no published reports regarding the use of psychostimulants for the control of deviant sexuality, despite the diagnosis of learning disabilities and attention deficit hyperactivity disorder in some male paraphiliacs.*'

I personally find this a very worrying statement as the writer has now drawn in those with learning difficulties and ADHD into this disturbing equation, positioning both groups among deviants because a small number have possibly similar habits. Why should anti-psychotics be used on either as the writer suggests they are? Equally disturbing, the writer admits that some treatment regimens cause paraphilia (a very strange term as employed here) in patients and a cocktail of drugs, sufficient to smother all thought and feeling, has proved effective in dealing with paraphilia in some cases. Given the effects, that should come as no surprise!

A review:

While devising different treatments for sexual predators and paedophiles and to then include sex between consenting adults within the paradigm of paraphilia is strange and worrying. Unfortunately, the writer has gained his understanding of paraphilia via DSM-5.

Mental health categories often function in this way, a category is identified and then expanded upon embracing, if in theory only, most of the population. The language employed in describing the (surely a multitude) suffering from this hypothesised category of mental illness feels like puritanism raising its mortified head. The DSM as a scientific text is based on hearsay not actuality[38]. Although the actions of certain people can be measured and observed, placing it within the parameters of mental health does not appear to help in any way except to provide work for psychiatrists. In our societies, psychiatry has a free hand with no real constraints other than the law courts.

---

[38] Post by Former NIMH Director Thomas Insel: Transforming Diagnosis *By **Thomas Insel** on April 29,*

13/https://www.nimh.nih.gov/about/directors/thomas-insel/blog/2013/transforming-diagnosis.shtml

In the context of this paper, leaving paedophilia within criminal parameters seems justified as thereby proper judgements based on law, not hypothesis, can be exercised identifying the different and differing forms of sexual behaviour itemised by the author and not asserting that they are all the same and that cross-dressing and promiscuity occupy the same moral and criminal perspective as paedophilia. Psychiatry occupies a separate, indeed competing, set of values to courts of law and seeks where possible to implement those values. Although adults in general are not allowed by law to act in certain ways towards children, locking them up, prescribing drugs, assuming guardianship, if a physician determines a child is mentally ill he or she can do fairly much whatever they like.

The writer appears to hold that *excess* implies mental imbalance, conflating different forms of behaviour that are very dissimilar in outcomes, whether that excess negatively affects others or not. The excess not the outcome informs his assessment of mental illness.

While the paper has concentrated on monoamine mechanisms it has done so only in a lessening of sexual feeling and increase of sexual feeling paradigm which in fact tends to be an illegal programme in the West, as the end result is castration. The author has gathered information solely on animal experiments but not on experiments focused on animals, like chimpanzees, which are biologically close to human beings. The use of experiments on rats leads to the observation: *have you ever seen a rat drive a car or catch a train to work each morning?* While again I can be accused of flippancy, modern psychiatry constructs its belief systems (the phrase is meant) on the basis that human beings have neither minds nor intelligence-excluding themselves of course from these observations. There is no suggestion in this paper that human beings possess intentionality, only the experimenter has that human trait.

The only treatment outcome provided appears to be a compound of chemicals strong enough to smoother the patient's feelings and actions, something noted by Joanna Moncrieff and her colleagues.

Lastly, there is no attempt here, nor will you find it elsewhere in psychiatric papers, to include actual ideas nor engage with other ideas or points of view. In one way, morally disreputable people (in Middle Americas viewpoint-DSM) are re-classified as mentally ill. Modern psychiatry, certainly since the rise of monoamine hypothesis, has become strikingly one dimensional in its approach while at the same time radically increasing the number of behaviours classified as mental illness and fragmenting such illnesses into separate ones. The writer (this is habitual) has not bothered to consult anthropology as a way of understanding human relationships, psychology, or a multitude of other possible disciplines. The writer has little apparent interest either in animal behaviour except within their sexual behaviour, with no interest in what may cause that behaviour. He and his colleagues have not it seems bothered to consult zoologists. Why do rats exhibit the sex life they do, cats and dogs, and can that throw any possible light on matters? Functioning within such a narrow spectrum when attempting to understand human behaviour seems highly irresponsible and arrogant. *A fundamental complaint with this approach is that no genuine understanding of the person and their actions is shown, only alteration of behaviour is considered. Such an approach has nothing to do with psychology, but has much to do with control and policing.*

PAPER 3:[39]

The point of this paper is not simply to engage with the Monoamine Hypothesis but also to throw light on psychiatric thinking. There is no implicit targeting of subject matter, but a random choice. The next paper to be analysed considers the connection between monoamine treatments and depression. This paper turned out to be a good example of the disease paradigm exclusively employed by psychiatrists until recently in that all forms of mental illness are the result of malfunctions in brain receptors and are not the consequence of stressful, difficult and negative environments or sudden difficult events such as failure in exams or the loss of relationships. Oddly, while taking this view psychiatry has gained its evidence from post-mortems but mainly through experiments on rats in which so-called depression has been induced through planned stress conditions in the laboratory.

The writer begins by making an epigrammatic statement, a style of writing common to psychiatry, asserting that in convoluted but clear sentences that the drugs most certainly work, and yet within the main text the language acknowledges the hypothesis status of the Monoamine Hypothesis. The writer judiciously employs 'belief', 'should', etc, to convey the tentative nature of his conclusions.

The paper than in rapid succession considers a conclusive range of activities established by the human neurone in processing or not processing serotonin. The processes are minute and itemised rigorously. Claims are made in rapid succession. 5-HT a serotonin is identified as an important element in neurosis in the over 50s, although it's other known affect is in the development of hyperthermia in rats. While the effects on rats are significant factors in the development of drugs depression is induced in the rats, and yet the paper, as with all such papers, fails to consider the difference to human long-term depression. Or if the rats' depression is exactly the same as human depression or simply a reaction to stress that dissipates once the stress is lifted. The two forms are related through observation and autopsy, but are they really the same? Nevertheless, he ends by stating that conclusions on his highly delineated activities of chemicals in the brain rest on assumptions, *and thereby meet hypothesis requirements, not that of proof.*

Several references to potential suicides or achieved suicides with increased $a2$ adrenergic receptors (443) and 5-HT 2A in teenage suicide victims nRMA levels for the receptors in the pre-frontal cortex (page 444) but not how it got there except it seems as the cause, unproven for the suicide. It might have arrived there as a consequence of events in the victims environments for example but this possibility is not explored or acknowledged. The abiding impression is that post-mortem provides the evidence on human victims but without situating any rationale for build ups of certain receptors. While these experiments on rats deliberately cause affective states in these animals, if that is what they were and not other responses, at no point does the writer infer or conclude that the same process might have occurred in the human victims, but treats the evidence in their brains as proof of the prevailing disease paradigm. Belief that the suicide victims were motivated by depression alone, appears to limit investigation into other possibilities. Many of my clients have reported on the feelings of suicide induced by prescribed drugs. The sense of being disconnected from world and Self caused by the drugs encourage feelings of alienation and despair. I have already had two cases

[39] Central monoamines and their role in major depressionS Abdalla Salem Elhwuegi Department of Pharmacology and Toxicology, Faculty of Pharmacy and Health Sciences, Ajman University of Sci

referred to me in Portugal with both repeating the same experiences-the drugs made them suicidal and altered their behaviour. Overall the writer decides that there are no contributory factors in teenage suicide but the end result of their depressive disease. The association between real or imaginary brain malfunction related to serotonin levels is maintained and no other possible cause considered.

As a consequence of this approach, patients are not communicated with in order to contribute to the psychiatrist's understanding, with professional retention of the distance required in General Hospitals, and functioning as if their own behaviour has no effect on patients. The inner life, doubts, worries, general concerns of the patient were ignored along with normal attitudes towards their own conduct. Treating people like objects has an effect on them. One client of mine was categorised while young, wrongly he felt, and was then subjected to appalling treatment by his family. None of this was factored into his increasingly depressed state, which was seen as a normal result of the disease he was suffering from. The professional's detachment from consequences means detachment from reality. The literature on psychotropic drugs is overwhelmingly from medical sources, with almost none from patients, except on internet sites where they can on occasion be found in profusion, almost all negative.[40]

This is a very technical paper but what emerges is 1) that depression is approached as a disease 2) patients are not identified within any context, they simply exist, nor does there appear any reason to discuss matters with them. The implication is that the patients had nothing to communicate about how they felt and why they felt the way they did, no more than someone suffering from measles can add to their treatment. 3) the evidence for the physicians paradigms come from human corpses and laboratory animals 4) *we know absolutely nothing about the patients and their subjective experiences, how they respond is ignored.*

In the end, we really only have physicians' word for the effectiveness of their treatments as no genuine evidence of success or failure is offered, merely assertions of efficacy. We hear from no other sources, certainly not the patients. No external or internal agency has checked or checks on their results. The whole matter of diagnosis, treatment and cure exists within a liminal (unreal) world in which the physician manages like a small-time autocrat and patients are both anonymous and passive, no more than treatment fodder. Assumptions are continually made on the efficacy of the treatments, and on the correctness of the monoamine paradigm with a surprising lack of corroborating evidence. Assumptions are indeed made about the rats suffering depression, which intuition suggests cannot be the same as human depression, human brains after all have greater emotional and cognitive complexity. At no point is this addressed. The human sufferers are not viewed as any different to the rats. As I remarked earlier, while depression in the laboratory animals is induced there are no visible debates on the possibility that human depression might be induced too, nor are any other possibilities considered. Joanne Moncrieff [41] suggests, given human variation, while some people are congenitally happy, others are congenitally sad. Here, we are again concerned with character not mental illness. Certainly some people clearly find it more difficult to overcome setbacks while others thrive on such things as listening to my clients such personality constructions can easily be developed over

[40] http://news.bbc.co.uk/1/high/health/1325629.stm
[41] The Psychoactive Effects of Psychiatric Medication: The Elephant in the Room Joanna Moncrieff M.B.B.S. , David Cohen & Sally Porter. 2013.A

time through abuse in the home or in the community. When I was a child abuse for example was rampant, individuals were likely to be bullied at home, school or work, driving many into depressive states. Drugs could not meet their needs, just exacerbate the problems.

Nevertheless, where is the science here, except as some kind of satire? Although the writer insists that there is considerable clinical and experimental evidence for the reliability of the monoamine hypothesis, the experiments have been done on depression induced (can rats really be depressed in the same fashion as human beings?) rats. What actual science is involved here? As I said above, there is no external agencies verifying the conclusions. As would be expected, research into rats indicate huge differences in brain functioning between rats and humans[42] but I have not yet found any reference to these differences in papers discussing monoamine efficacy or the efficacy of psychotropic drugs.[43] This is all very poor science indeed![44]

The only science that seems involved is clinical observation, if they can really be said to be a science. A professional collects data on the treatment they or a colleague provides, notes are made. This seems to be the only information gathering and learning process. The skills of the professional are elemental in this approach, but it does not concern the legitimacy of treatment but that of approach. The authenticity of treatments is not thereby challenged nor the capabilities of the professional. It functions therefore as a reinforcement technique confirming already held ideas.

Nevertheless, there is one scientific method, deductionism, being used, with reference to a well-known syllogism:

Psychiatrists treat people

Treating people is good

Therefore psychiatric treatments are good.

This can be applied thereby to monoamine hypothesis simply enough.

Psychiatry is one of the most successful models of psychophysical reductionism, whereby psychological phenomenon is reduced to its physical and chemical components centred on the reduction of patients. The patients, human beings, are reduced to little more than ciphers without minds, intelligence or potential. They are merely diseases. In this fashion, it is easy thereby to conflate patients with animals and objectify them. Psychiatry, with respect to this theory, bypasses functionalism by eliminating the functions of the patient through the disease model further reducing them to objects of experimentation and direct products of the doctor.

---

[42] Post by Former NIMH Director Thomas Insel: insel/blog/2013/transforming Diagnosis *By Thomas Insel* on April 29, 2013/ https://www.nimh.nih.gov/about/directors/thomas2013.A
[43] Savanna, Stephane. Can Rats Reason? Psychology of Consciousness: Theory, Research and Practice. 2015. Vol 2. No 4. 404-429.
[44] Hughes, Cohen, Johnson. Adverse event assessment methods in published trials of psychotropic drugs: Poor reporting and neglect of emerging safety concerns. International Journal of Risk and Safety In Medicine 28 (2016) 101-1014.

The patient's identity is subsumed within the disease they model (not represent) as the active component is the disease.

Psychiatry appears to believe that the mind is reducible to processes within the brain related to the activity of numerous reception, transmission and trigger systems, producing thereby a belief in the independent and at the same time the unified operation of mood triggers. The proficiency of all or a large number of neurons indicates mental health, defined through psychiatric understandings, based on the patient relationship to physician and the patient's relationship to psychotropic drugs. The patient and the psychiatrist inhabit a dialectic between mental health and illness determined by the physician and not it seems negotiated by the patient. Experiences such as art, pleasure, writing, internally and externally are eliminated from patient's internal and external relationships. Common concepts of the mind are eliminated.

Assessment:

Working in the area of mental health for a few years, I was intrigued by the contrasting views of those in receipt of treatment and those giving it, particularly the effects of psychotropic drugs. I began listening to patients and making thereby comparisons with papers on the Lancet and in various journals. They seemed diametrically opposed.

A) **My own assessment over many years revealed that prescription psychotropic drugs had a number of clear, observable effects:**

1) Long term dependency

2) Somnambulant attributes, inexpressive features and voice tone.

3) Encouraged and determined slowing of movement, cognition and ambition.

4) Encouraged and even initiated psychological turmoil.

5) Created or increased depression in a number of clients.

6) Initiated suicidal thoughts.

7) Created feelings of alienation

8) Created inability to connect to others, and lead to psychopathic tendencies and fantasies that occasionally were acted out.

9) In a number of cases personality disorder.

10) Created a diminishment of artistic expression

11) Diminished achievement levels

12) Could in some cases create paranoia

13) Produced outbursts of anger

14) Possible acrophobia

Such noticeable and noted effects increased with length of use.

B) From a child social worker's observations of working with children diagnosed with mental illness:

What is the process of diagnosing a disorder then? The concept of disorder is a cut-off point, a threshold, above which the symptoms in question are considered to cause serious suffering and impairment. Because resilience factors vary individually, this threshold should also vary individually. Diagnosis, on the other hand, is purely a construct. It is a cluster of symptoms out of which a person needs to present a certain number of them during a certain period of time in order to be diagnosed, that is, classified. The symptoms referred to have an interesting characteristic in common: they are all externally observed.

For instance, let's imagine that during four weeks I present fever and digestive problems. The symptoms and the length of time are enough to diagnose me with the "Stomach-ache disorder". However, a simple test and/or a painful internal examination would have clarified that I had either an allergy to some kind of food or a stomach cancer. Two very different conditions that presented some similar symptoms; the symptoms that did not coincide were not recorded since they were not included in the diagnostic criteria for the disorder. If we do not tolerate this approach with our stomach, why we do so with our brain? ADHD claims to imply a change in brain structures, yet no brain scan is taken to make the diagnose. We know that people under prolonged conditions of trauma and/or stress will experience eventually some physiological changes, such as an increased heart rate even at rest, yet no looked after child is checked on this regardless of their life histories.

In addition, psychiatric diagnosis, particularly in children and adolescents, takes de meaning of a symptom a little bit further. In the example above, I went to my GP because I felt pain in my stomach. My condition is diagnosed following my account of my experience. Yet, in children and adolescent's mental health, the account that is most often heard is that one of the adults surrounding them. At a time when nobody doubts the value of listening to children's voices is worth considering how much a diagnose of ODD, for example, actually reflects the life experienced from the child's point of view.

Besides these more medical considerations, there are also others. We cannot ignore the fact that to diagnose somebody with a mental health disorder is a process akin to diagnose with an illness. That is, the condition lies within the person-patient. This process completely downplays the causal influence played by the social and developmental contexts. When we design a preventive treatment for the flu, for example, we are looking for a vaccine. Yet when we design a preventive intervention for these mental health disorders, we need to look at aspects such as living and work conditions or support networks. In the flu case it is easy to implement; we all know that the flu symptoms are caused by a virus. It is practically impossible to implement in the case of the mental health disorders, where all our interventions are directed to minimise the symptoms, not to end with their cause, because we simply do not talk about their cause. Only the diagnose of PTSD includes a cause in its criteria. This despite the fact of the increasing number of studies starting to link social issues such as poverty (see Wilkinson and Pickett) or childhood maltreatment (see Keyes et al.) to mental health disorders.[45]

[45]Fernandez, Ana olea. PSYCHIATRIC DIAGNOSIS & PSYCHOTROPIC DRUGS IN LOOKED AFTER CHILDREN &

The drug-based construct of mental illness, formed upon generic descriptions based on observation with symptoms interpreted exclusively by physicians, have provided modern archetypes –personality disorder, narcissism, psychosis- placing patients within an eternal present and eliminating causation, such as childhood abuse. Personality Disorder resembles cartoon stick figures of human actors. Although there have been noted changes, the disease based model has, it appears, both eliminated the mind (with regard to patients) and extended greater control over patient's lives.

C) **Effects on individual personalities by prescribed drugs seems little different from the effects of a variety of psychotropic drugs from tobacco, coffee to cocaine.**

Summing up:

1) The research has been mainly restricted to animals, particularly rats, but little work seems to have been done on the validity, let alone veracity, of transposing research focused on one kind of mammal of comparatively reduced complexity onto the most complex of mammals. The psychiatric profession has on this basis convinced itself of the authenticity of both their paradigms and treatments.

2) Apart from the apparent evidence accrued from experimentation on rats (not exclusively), post-mortem evidence has been sought from suicide victims. While Elhwuegi (Paper 3) declares in his short conclusion that post-mortem evidence has proved the monoamine hypothesis this is absolutely denied in a recent thorough research (Klimeka, Robersona, et al: Serotonin transporter and MAO-B levels in monoamine nuclei of the human brainstem are normal in major depression)[46] into the matter. The authors impose reservations, but their conclusions are clear. No matter all the exhaustive preamble, the location of proteins, receptors within a trigger paradigm, there actually is no genuine evidence.

The present study is the first anatomically detailed examination of the serotonergic innervation of the human noradrenergic LC, providing a thorough evaluation of serotonin input to multiple levels of the LC along its rostro-caudal axis. In addition, the possibility that innervation of the LC by serotonergic terminals may be abnormal in major depression was investigated for the first time. The results of this study demonstrate a moderate innervation of the human LC by serotonin neurons that is organized evenly throughout the LC. However, based on two markers of serotonergic innervation (MAO-B and SERT), no evidence of an altered serotonergic input to the LC in major depression was observed.

Research reservations:
Since major depression is a complex disease process, several neurotransmitter systems including norepinephrine, dopamine and serotonin, as well as multiple brain regions,

---

[46] Journal of Psychiatric Research 37 (2003) 387-397.

are likely to be significantly involved. Given the physiological integration of monoaminergic systems in the brain and their potential involvement in the neurochemical pathology of depression (Ordway et al., 2002), one can conceive of a pathophysiology of depression that would not, on theoretical grounds, require that all proteins will be abnormal in their relevant psychobiological domains. The study of other markers of serotonergic innervation of the LC, as well as serotonin receptor-linked second messenger systems, should be undertaken before concluding that serotonergic modulation of the LC is normal in major depression.

3) The experiments on animals involves induced depression, but there seems no debate within psychiatry on whether or not rats' responses can thereby truly be identified as depression. Nor is there any expressed concern about the apparent latent depression of human patients and the induced depression of animals.

4) Rats' brains are substantively and substantially different to human brains. Savanah[47] mentions the dual psychology of human beings, absent, as one might expect in rats, and if, as must at present be assumed, rats lack self-consciousness how do these factors affect comparison, if any can reliably be made at all? A rat's *depression* would not be self-referential but human depression would with layers of reference unlikely in a rat. Would that effect monoamine activity? No one asks. As science this is all very poor indeed.

5) Psychiatric construction of the mind, based on extremely crude reductionism, seems rarely to be challenged. In fact the psychiatric model fits neatly into a top-down approach and treatment with drugs. Counsellors and psycho-therapists have a far more complex model.

6) Not touched on here, but considered by Joanne Moncrieff and David Cohen, et al, in their important paper *'The Elephant in the Room'*, [48]is the one way exploration of mental illness through an effusion of clinical propaganda. I recently saw a drama on TV about a country doctor who had to deal with a young student suffering from psychosis (sic). The student was acting remarkably odd because he had chosen to stop taking his drugs. A small matter, but dealing with a wide range of mental health sufferers, I never saw this once concluding it was a physicians' myth to provide an explanation for the actual functioning of psychotropic drugs, which is that the effects wear off. A function they deny. Nevertheless, look into any magazine, newspaper, etc, and you will see the medical model discussed there as scientific truth-monoamine hypothesis is proven (it is not), psychotropic drugs are a modern miracle (they are not), the range of psychiatric diagnosis is scientifically based (it is not). Many definitions of mental illness in DSM-5 are simply social prejudice.

7) This paper has hopefully focused some light on psychiatry's claims for scientific authenticity and credibility and found them wanting. Experiments and research into

[47]Savanna, Stephane. <u>Can Rats Reason</u>? Psychology of Consciousness: Theory, Research and Practice. 2015. Vol 2. No 4. 404-429.

[48] The Psychoactive Effects of Psychiatric Medication: The Elephant in the Room Joanna Moncrieff M.B.B.S. , David Cohen & Sally Porter. 2013.A

psychiatric truths, such as monoamine hypothesis and the efficacy of drugs, are deeply flawed with simple questions not being asked, checks not being done rigorously and a lack of an overarching authority to ferret through and into psychiatric ideas and practices to weigh their authenticity.

For example, Personality Disorder as a scientific category leaves a great deal to be desired and is a matter of contention and concern.[49] The use of psychiatric categories based on social prejudice within DSM-5, provides support for worrying over this most uncertain of all *sciences*.

8) Possible effects on patient's health through long term or excessive use: *Sudden death of cardiac origin and psychotropic drugs.* Quadirri Timour, et al. Frontiers in Pharmacology. 10 May 2012. Doi: 10.3389/fphar.2012.0008

Possible genetic damage due to long-term exposure tp psychotropic drugs. Topinka, et al. Psychiatric Research Unit, Prague.

---

[49] Gotzschc-Astrup, Oluf/Moskowitz, Andrew. Personality Disorders and the DSM-5: scientific and extra-scientific factors in the maintenance of the status quo. Australian and New Zealand Journal of Psychiatry.

Personality Disorder, Truth and Deceit.

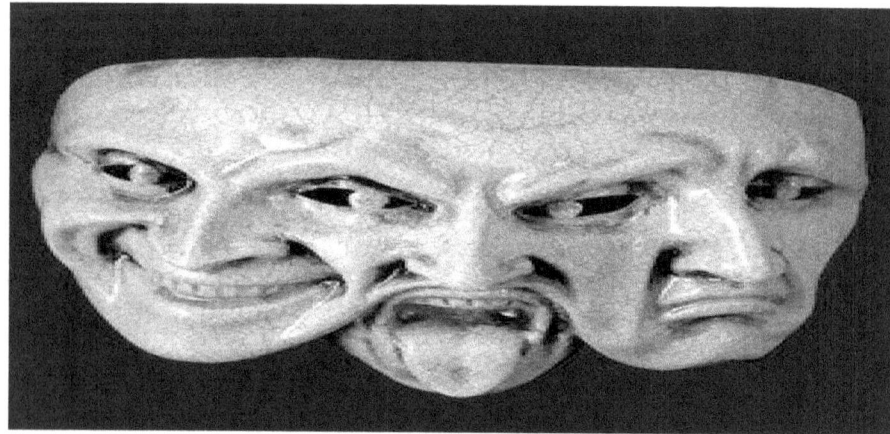

Archetypes: Masks: Personality Disorder?

Personality disorders are rarely seen as a form of mental illness but nevertheless at the same time are regularly claimed as the preserve of psychiatry. Sufferers from this disorder (sic) have been for example referred to as anti-social types, but without any further examination or apparent understanding of the properties of society, its strategies of conformity. It is a diagnosis in which physician subjectivity plays a considerable part inviting social and gender prejudice to function under the guise of clinical judgement. The debate on its illness' status has in fact been resolved by on the one hand saying it is not an illness, and many do, and on the other grasping it as a clinical problem-in other words the preserve of doctors. [50] The regular publication of the DSM (*The Diagnostic and Statistical Manual of Mental Disorders-5*) and the claims appended to it as a scientific document (sic) have given the upper hand to the latter, but with continued protests from the former.

I have again, as before, chosen the paper attached to this essay P*ersonality Disorder in Perspective*[51] at random. While this can be considered inappropriate by some, in fact one psychiatric paper closely resembles another, and this is especially so in the case of papers proving the validity of the monoamine hypothesis, each of which could have been written by a computer. Indeed '*Advances in the classification, epedimiology, treatment and prognosis of personality disorders shows personality disorders are common, extensive in their pathology, and cause much suffering* ' (Tyrer, et al) It is with these kind of testimonies in mind that the

[50]Tyrer, Casey, Ferguson Personality Disorder in Perspective.. The British Journal of Psychiatry. 1991. 159: Page 1.

[51] Tyrer, Casey, Ferguson. Personality Disorder in Perspective. British Journal of Psychiatry. 1991.159. 463-471

claims will be considered, attempting to discover if the above criterion are met and in the process attempting to unravel whether or not scientific methods are being employed.

In order to investigate the authenticity of the classification, whether or not psychiatrists are justified in using it or in actually involving themselves with people considered to be suffering from these conditions, I will consider the views of a variety of commentators but predominantly the paper mentioned above by Tyrer, et al, Roy Porter, Michel Foucault, Pinel, and Philippe Huneman. It has to be acknowledged that the general population receives ideas on personality disorder from the medical profession, usually considered a trusted and uncorrupted source, and yet is it possible that the matter is not quite so straightforward? While I understand that people believe the medical profession these papers assert that the science behind their beliefs is often deeply flawed and that unfortunately they are rarely challenged and critiqued. Unlike many hypothesis, medical ones can be acted upon without the accompanying proof (monoamine hypothesis and psychotropic drugs) and with the collusion, indeed encouragement, of the state.

This paper will consider throughout the nature of archetypes (on which Personality Disorder is based), descriptions of human personality in often one dimensional aspects that in both their clinical and diagnostic functions cannot be viewed as scientific, the growth of hospitals and the consequent effect on the appearance of psychiatry, Pinel's methods and written work and the effects of these on the construction of physician power and authority.

1.

Personality disorders do not inhabit a mental state, they do not replicate any of the properties of schizophrenia or mania but are mainly concerned with attitude and behaviour. They have according to Tyrer, Casey and Ferguson[52] been recorded by various writers for thousands of years, initially [53] by the Greek philosopher Theothrastus who described thirty Athenian characters, each of which Tyrer et al claim represent personality disorders. The commentators have neglected to mention, if they were actually aware of it, that the character sketches are not clinical in nature but simply sketches demonstrating types reflecting the archetypal-based comedies of the day. In effect, it is as if the writers had employed Dickens' Mr Pecksniff or Fagin as evidence for medical conditions, omitting to mention that a writer made them up to add depth and energy to a novel. Theothrastus' compositions had a literary function and were designed to provide material for the new comedy of the age.[54] This is indicative of the writers approach to knowledge, common with writings on psychiatry that rarely engage with other forms of knowledge.

The introduction to the 1902 translation [55] references literary characters or archetypes, not true ones: The Flatterer, The Avaricous man, The Braggart, The Pompous Man, The Boor, The

---

[53] Most commentators in these areas tend to have limited knowledge of the past but nevertheless constantly reference it to prove points.

[54] The writers do not allude to this, in fact seem unaware of their literary function.

[55] The Characters of Theophrastus A 'Translation^ with Introduction By Charles E. Bennett and William A. Hammond Professors in Cornell University Longmans, Green,

Gross Man, types for an audience to immediately recognise and laugh over. It is such literary constructs that the writers claim influential psychological judgements have been built on. The writers have confused literary techniques with reality. Is it indeed possible that the DSM is informed by such thinking?

The next evidence they produce is generalised, insisting that many other past cultures also provided evidence of personality disorders but as they fail here to include any such examples their assertion cannot be challenged. In world culture there has been at various times use made of archetypal characters to express ideas. This can be seen in Ancient Sumerian culture-the gods for example and demi-gods-Hebrew literature-Samson is identified as having strength and not provided with many other traits, Jezebel is the archetype of female paganism-but these are literary techniques to create meaning. Even complex characters such as Gilgamesh explore certain traits. Gilgamesh could realistically be used to explore depression through loss, but the actual lessons to be learned are much deeper and beyond the parameters of psychiatry. They include dealing with identity, the responsibilities of extreme power and human beings relationship to the gods. In fact, psychiatry's understanding of human nature is essentially one dimensional, indeed deeply superficial. Paradigms of intellectual and spiritual despair are reduced to archetypal tropes with meaning only to psychiatry itself. As this paper hopes to prove, they are both unreal and unsubstantiated. Nevertheless, as archetypes are representative, used as symbols and metaphors, they can and do throw a light on psychiatric thought processes.

For Carl Jung archetypes[56] were the triggers for energy, and were appropriate as fundamental elements of human personality in relation to other complementary or conflicting archetypes-human beings had complexes not disorders. The psychiatric model gives human beings single archetypes to inhabit with nothing more, such as paranoid, obsessive-but these are not then balanced out as they are in human beings with other archetypes. In Jung's model they are expressed in greater complexity within ideas such as anima, shadow, and wise child, all mingled where appropriate. Therefore in Jung's psychology the paranoid archetype might be balanced out with father archetype, providing therefore depth. The shadow archetype, perhaps closest to the paranoia archetype of psychiatry, provides a rounded understanding of human motivations through being expressed via other archetypes. Jingis Khan, while expressed as a murderous, brutal conqueror was also a wise administrator and father. Jung's version of human beings is positive and not overwhelmed by problems. In psychiatry, people are identified through one archetype, which tends to be negative. Personality Disorder, unlike human personality in general has few if any positives projecting onto patients and outward to interested readers like the different masks of stage villains. Psychiatric archetypes are situated in an everlasting present with only a nod to aetiology, *unchanging and unchangeable except through psychiatry (see below on Huneman's analysis of Pinel.)* While Jung's archetypes are expressed through myth and metaphor as part of a collective unconscious, psychiatric archetypes are

and Co. 91 and 93 Fifth Avenue, New York London and Bombay 1902.
http://www.archive.org/stream/charactersoftheo00theorich/charactersoftheo00theoric
h_djvu.txt
[56] Archetypes and the Collective Unconscious (Collected Works of C.G. Jung) Princeton University Press. 1969.

expressions of *'mental illness'*-the energy this engenders. Therefore, they are the metaphor. Are they also the myth behind psychiatry's desire for expansion?

Pinel: the first psychiatrist?

Finally, Tyrer et al, arrive at Philippe Pinel, a physician in Revolutionary France and the first apparent mental health clinician, who became *physician of infirmeries* at Bicetre, a hospital for men in Paris. As with many similar establishments of the time it functioned as workhouse/prison/and general depository for unwanted male citizens. Later he ran the women's hospital of Salpetrietre, also in Paris that served the same purpose. He immediately put the daemonic aetiology of mental illness aside so legend has it (although the treatments he championed were already employed in Britain for example),[57] released the insane from their chains, and provided a clinical, descriptive approach to mental illness. In fact most of the achievements attributed to Pinel belonged to Jean-Baptiste Pussin, the superintendent of Bicetre mental ward, and his wife, Marguerite. Pinel learnt from both and they gave him immense support in his researches. He took Pussin, who had no scientific or academic qualifications, with him to Salpetrietre as a special assistant. It was Pussin who began the process, utilised by Pinel, of making observations and taking down notes on patients.

Pinel meanwhile noted, for example, *that: "being held in esteem, having honour, dignity, wealth, fame, which though they may be factitious, always distressing and rarely fully satisfied, often give way to the overturning of reason". He spoke of avarice, pride, friendship, bigotry, the desire for reputation, for conquest, and vanity.*[58] In the difficult circumstances of the time, it is not possible to ascertain the appropriateness of his approach here, except that he does not seem to mention poverty for example although he wrote of stress as a reason for mental illness. Pinel appears to have understood human suffering and frustration through the personality not circumstances, reflecting present day psychiatric perspectives. The list of contributing traits presented above are moral in nature, pride, as presented in comedies based on type, considered a viable aetiology.

Although Pinel did not invent Moral Treatment (Management), which had already been developed by the Pussins consisting in part of treating patients with respect and kindness, releasing them from their chains, and talking with them about their conditions, combating delusions for example with quiet, persuasive rationality, he nevertheless wrote important work championing their methods and providing rationales for their successes and conclusions on their and his observations. In 1801 he wrote the *Treatise on Insanity* and later his *Memoirs on Madness.* In Britain, William Tuke was developing the same methods at The Retreat, a private

---

[57] MacKenzie, Charlotte. Psychiatry For the Rich, A History of Ticehurst Private Asylum, 1792-1917. Routledge, London-New York. 1992: page 6.
[58] Moral Treatment: Philippe Pinel
Mrs. Sushma. C1*, Dr. Meghamala. S. Tavaragi2The International Journal of Indian Psychology ISSN 2348-5396 (e) | ISSN: 2349-3429 (p) Volume 3, Issue 2, No.8, DIP: 18.01.153/20160302 ISBN: 978-1-329-95395-6
http://www.ijip.in | January - March, 2016

facility in York.[59] Although it meant various things, inculcating reason, a particular bugbear of Foucault[60], back into a mad person was an important element.

One of Pinel's goals appears to have been the creation of a separate profession of mental health doctor or alienist. Although alienists existed, certainly in Britain, these tended to be unqualified and working in private establishments. While Tuke preserved a hands on approach with his patients, Pinel stood apart, observed and made notes.[61] Such a separation ensured, by its nature, distorted communication as all communication between doctor and patient was re-ordered by the doctor. By then taking notes, only the doctor's thoughts and voice were and are visible.

2. Hospitals:

In France and in Britain the construction of hospitals changed the doctor/patient dichotomy. [62]Not only were doctors in a more intimate relationship with patients, allowing for closer examination of illness, they also controlled the environment that patients were in. Hospitals became, certainly in time, the physician's kingdom or manorial estate where they formed reality and in the process controlled day to day perceptions. [63] Pinel developed care methodology with the mentally ill that played a leading part in establishing the ensuing hierarchy of the mental health services through a number of administrative and diagnostic innovations within French Hospitals. He created a professional ideological template that is still with us, procedures and diagnosis dependent on identifiable single phrases that once written time could not be adjusted, or not by much.

Both the Bicetre and Salpetrietre were part of the French General Hospital institutions formed by the Kings of the 17th and 18th century. When Pinel arrived at Bicetre he separated the mentally ill from the rest of the residents, prostitutes, vagrants, criminals and vagrants, thereby, according to Foucault[64], creating the division between normal and abnormal, making the mentally ill in a dichotomy to normal people, whatever that may have meant, which represented a hierarchy with physicians at the top. Psychiatrists were and are the most rationale of all, but without abnormality there can be no normality.

Foucault's argument[65], although it has merit in describing physician control of the constructs of mental illness and the environments in which they were then contained, fails otherwise as, a

---

[59] Digby, Anne. Madness, Orality and Medicine. A Study of the York Retreat, 1796-1914. Cambridge University Press. 1985.

[60]https://monoskop.org/images/1/14/Foucault_Michel_Madness_and_Civilization_A_History_of_Insanity_in_t he_Age_of_Reason.pdf

[61] Digby, Anne. Orality and Medicine...

[62] A Social History of Madness. Stories of the Insane. Weidenfeld & Nicolson. 1987: p 167.

[63] Madness, Morality and Medicine. A Study of the York Retreat, 1796-1914. Cambridge University Press. 1985: page 3.

[64]tps://monoskop.org/images/1/14/Foucault_Michel_Madness_and_Civilization_A_History_of_Insanity_in_th e_Age_of_Reason.pdf

[65]https://monoskop.org/images/1/14/Foucault_Michel_Madness_and_Civilization_A_History_of_Insanity_in_t he_Age_of_Reason.pdf

point already made, in Britain private mental hospitals had long existed. The Great Incarceration noted by Foucault occurred mainly in France as a consequence of Louis XIV's absolutism of the 17th century, and in Britain, according to Roy Porter[66] decentralisation occurred instead. Stronger arguments here concern academics unravelling of the nature of the hospital and its impact on medicine, particularly psychiatry. An environment was created for the provision of a new group of professional medical administrators, whose rule over their patients became absolute. They, and often they alone, decided their patient's identity, perceptions and fates. When Pinel designed the structure of the mental hospital in France he also designed its ideology, whereby as Foucault more correctly remarks, physician authority and power was paramount. Its possibly earlier development in Britain[67] can be seen in conjunction with the later story of John Percival and the growth in professional claims and absolutism of alienists/psychiatrists. Percival, a patient at Brislington Hall run by Edward Long Fox, complained about the dominant ideology of the alienists who considered a patient sane if they fitted their conception of normality, one criterion being not showing negative emotion. If the patient remained obedient and obeyed the doctor, they were more likely to be judged sane than if they argued and were rebellious. [68]This fitted in with the ideology of Moral Training, whereby the physician was teaching patients to abandon flaws (see above) of pride, sloth, etc. The recovery of the patient was directly connected to the degree they obeyed the physician. This paper will demonstrate that similar thinking permeates modern psychiatry's notions of Personality Disorder-that is, not only is conformity necessary, but the pressures towards conformity come from a puritanical source.

Pinel's reputation and his understanding of mental illness reside within the *Traite medico-philosophique sur I'alienation mentale ou la manie* in which he states his nostology, the book that legend has it effectively introduced rationale psychiatry. Pinel examined many of the concepts of modern psychiatry, such as mania, and largely rejected somatic diseases and delirious fevers. Aside from the above criticisms, Foucault challenged the idea of Pinel as the liberator of the mentally ill, but insisted instead that he forged new chains. By separating the mad from the destitute and prostitutes, Pinel was not merely saying the mad were essentially different, but in doing so he established a separate class of expertise, creating its ideology and providing stable work for himself and other alienists. If the mad were different from normal people, only specialists could possibly understand them and also they needed to be in specialist care. The business model approach, itemised by Roy Porter and Andrew Scull, the present doyen of medical historians, will be dealt with in another paper.

Quite rightly, Foucault points out that patients became closely linked to the physician and their moral superiority-and supposition of intellectual superiority. Psychiatrists' sense of superiority can be overwhelming more so given the mechanistic learning factors involved in acquiring psychiatric knowledge! The arrangement gave psychiatrists immense power over patients, which they enjoy today, it is in fact a highly unusual powe. George III's doctor, Francis Willis

---

[66] A Social History of Madness. Stories of the Insane. Weidenfeld & Nicolson. 1987: p 167.
[67] A Social History of Madness. Stories of the Insane. Weidenfeld & Nicolson. 1987: p 167.
[68] An Unusual Power: Madhouses: Sane or Insane?

is a case in point. Roy Porter concludes here (1987: p 19) that this involved reclaiming the mad through the mad- *'personal charisma, force of character and individually designed inventive psychological strategies, of which one noted example was a form of hypnotism. '* Willis meanwhile held that the doctor's will could dominate the patient, and should to effect a cure. In the end, the evidence suggests he used violence against the vulnerable king.

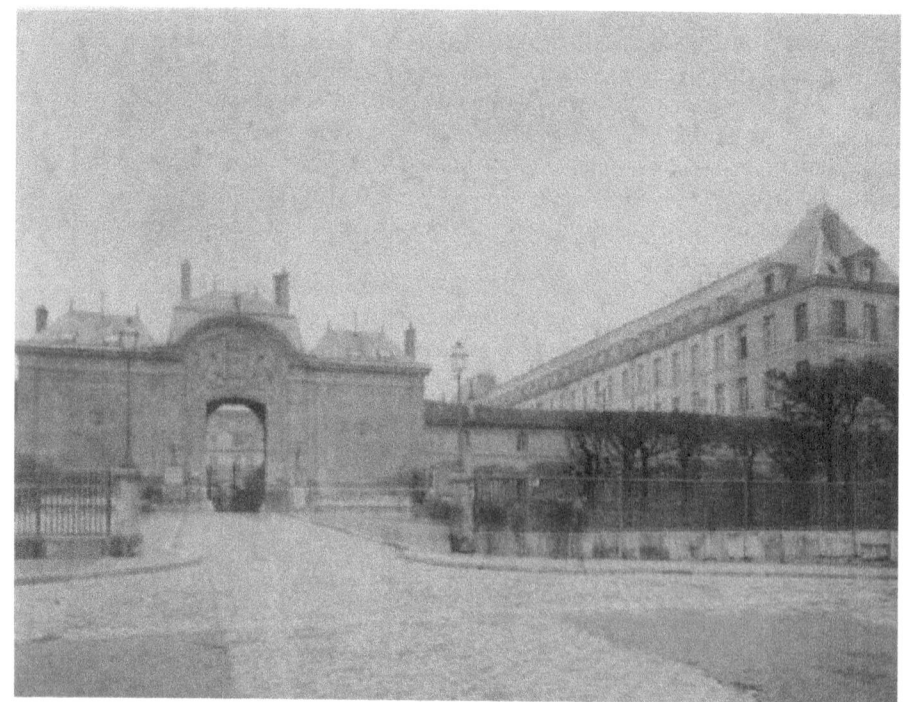

Bicetre Hospital

3. Pinel's writing, thinking and its effects:

Pinel's *Traite* is constructed of long case studies rather than just an elaboration of his theories. His case studies, like Freud's are short stories on the events in a person's life that may have precipitated (or not) their mental illness, and what occurs after treatment. Like Freud's cases, Pinel's are his view of another's narrative, not theirs, so as a story teller he controls what the reader knows. Like Freud, he selects aspects of the narrative, excluding other matters from the reader's understanding of events. The cases are not thereby a true record of events, only what Pinel decides the reader should know. The narrative shows a deviation from the normal, not healthy or well people, but those the narrator determines are not well and healthy and the perceptions the writer similarly concludes are not normal and healthy.

In these pages, Pinel constructed the nostology of pathological perceptions and behaviour, as well as describing and promoting the therapeutic practices involved. Philippe Huneman[69] shows that these cases determine the universal (a given pathology) and the individual, between the level of the visible at which symptoms take place and the invisible level of these symptoms as signifiers and whatever aetiology is used to explain the invisible. Thereby a patient with mania (?) or observed as such, describes their own condition by behaviour recognised by the physician from earlier descriptions. The physician further notes the new patient's behaviour, connecting the resultant description to other patients' behaviour who have received a diagnosis of mania. Alternatively, it can be seen as a patient seeing a doctor who references a list of behaviour/symptoms alongside of which is a description, as in the DSM, and the *patient becomes the description-or diagnosis*. Whichever view is taken, it is the doctor who decides what the patient is suffering from and neither the patient nor anyone else who knows the patient has a say in the matter. The doctor's procedures are absolute. Part of the myth perpetuated by psychiatry is that through observation they can understand and judge the internal workings of a patient; their understanding coalescing with understanding of the archetype or group.

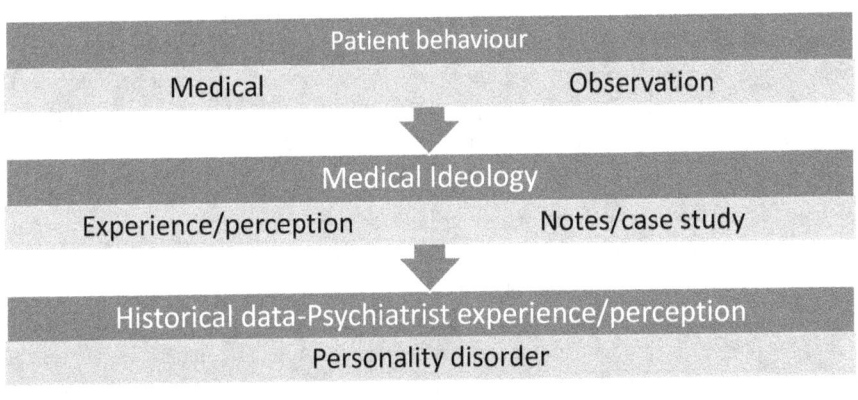

Clinical judgement distorts reality, not informs it.

In the example above, while the first patient the doctor sees might in fact have the mania his/her behaviour suggests they have, going by pre-determining descriptions and behaviour, the second patient might have a fever, be suffering food poisoning, been up all night with a screaming baby, or be overseeing a failing business. As only observation is employed as a diagnostic tool and, like Pinel, as the doctor does not communicate equally with the patient they do not and cannot know the patient's individual rationale. Whatever rationale the patient possesses has

---

[69] Writing the case-Pinel as Psychiatrist. Institute of Histoire et de Philosophie des Sciences et des Techniques, CNRS/Universite Paris I Sorbonne.

always to be subordinate to the doctor's rationale. This kind of approach is still employed today, and cannot remotely be considered scientific. It is considered scientific by psychiatrists on the logical basis that as psychiatrists are members of a science, their methods must at all times also be scientific.

Personality disorder as a paradigm:

Philippe Huneman,[70] who has analysed at length both Pinel's texts and ideas, demonstrates how Pinel's case study, as literature as well as performance, affected the development of psychiatry, its practices and ideologies-in this instance personality disorders as a paradigm. Huneman agrees that the development of psychiatry as a specialism went hand in hand with the development of the hospital as a place of cure as well as hospitality. Within the hospital the individual patient represents a statistical relationship between an individual, see above, and a group-the mad/mentally ill/or those with personality disorders. The patient becomes the statistic or description and the number losing thereby their humanity and becoming part of an archetype.

While Freud also controlled both narrative and perception of the patient's experiences, like psychiatrists he described and ordered his and their experiences and perceptions-that is he decided both nature and aetiology of experience through the processes of treatment. Freud acted not as a manager, like psychiatrists, but as an explorer or investigator. When I first began studying psychiatric writings, a long time ago, I read a compilation of case studies on the effects of masturbation on mental stability written in the 1950s and 1960s, which as literature I considered absorbing but as science implausible. When reading essays or articles on monoamine hypothesis or other current theories I get the same sense of entering a liminal world that is to one degree or another detached from the physical world.

In his *Memoirs on Madness*, Pinel demonstrates that faced with up to 200 patients he needed to sort them initially in his own mind, so to do that he employed rational relationships or categories. Huneman (page 6) connects this with methods associated with hospitals as institutions, separating people in pathological groups in order to treat them within those groups, and, as in the present day, in large numbers. Symptoms *appeared* to be shared, at least on the superficial level of physician observation. In pure medicine, Huneman holds, the clinical case as a discursive category creates order, or apparent order, out of confusion. *Taxonomies are ways of re-constructing reality, not indicators of reality –at least where measurable phenomenon is not available.* Every patient can be fitted into a box that resembles other boxes based on a few shared characteristics provided with a single treatment, usually drugs. He describes it as an intermediary position between *first impressions* and taxonomy, perfectly describing the nature of diagnosis-at best a useful but inadequate tool that functions for the benefit of the doctor and for the efficient running of the hospital or any other appropriate institution.

---

[70] Writing the case-Pinel as Psychiatrist. Institute of Histoire et de Philosophie des Sciences et des Techniques, CNRS/Universite Paris I Sorbonne.

These methods reflect those then being developed within physical diseases. The variable nature of individual expressions of illness represents an overall whole. In a plague symptoms may, with only minor variations, resemble each other denoting a common cause. We now know that in the past many plagues or illnesses were lumped together when often they were separate phenomenon. Pinel, we are informed (Huneman) introduced changes to the classical nostology by including case history, with less emphasis on phenomenological evidence. Not now so much the case, as looking for evidence in corpses is now de rigor in psychiatry-mainly to prove hypothesis. There is an obsession within psychiatric research of both proving and confirming overarching hypothesis-the effects of SSRIs on this problem or another. Developing a different nostology, Pinel thereby developed a medical specialism with declared differences to the physical nostology. He was creating psychiatry as an autonomous tradition in a sense appropriating or accommodating Moral Management (treatment) under his own procedures-'*its own objects, its own modes of intervention, an its own territory*' (Huneman). He gave to alienism a professional basis, providing it with the first steps towards status and credibility (page 8).

Before the British moral treatment innovators and Pinel there was only the abysmal hospital/prison/workhouses of France and Britain, and also the private mental homes in Britain run mainly by charlatans and fraudsters. Colin Jones[71] writes of the ease in which unwanted relatives had been imprisoned in mental hospitals, although laws had been put in place to prevent it. On page 377, he considers the *dissolute* daughters of '*honest*' citizens in a house for reforming prostitutes against their wishes. Ideas of reform and moral treatment were closely allied. This persuading of psychiatry to take on unwanted relatives under the pretence of mental instability went on in my direct experience only twenty years ago under the umbrella of personality disorder-an uncertain and unreliable definition. According to Jones (377) all a family had to do was turn up at a mental hospital with a letter from a Bishop and their relative would be taken in or detained. The impress of morality is clear and obvious.

When educated people, principally medical doctors, entered the arena to run the homes, creating salaries, careers and status, they sought credibility. They had to make treatment of the insane professional, with ideologies and specific treatment methodologies. People like Tuke and Pinel provided that with physician distance and observation techniques. Credibility was mainly established through managerial activity in asylums, and continued that way although psychiatrists claimed superlative knowledge of the mentally ill, and still do, their main role was control or management of the mentally ill. The knowledge was mainly, and remains, a façade. In the same way that the monoamine hypothesis provided the psychiatric profession with scientific credibility, so asylums provided them with credibility and monthly salaries.

Although, this was a time when many people who were not insane found themselves in French hospitals as a last resort, Pinel makes no mention of this tendency, see above, and seems to

---

[71] The Treatment of the Insane in eighteenth-and early nineteenth-century Montpelier. A Contribution to the Prehistory of the lunatic asylum in Provincial France. Medical History, 1980., 24: 371-390.

regard anyone in the mental wards as insane. As they were presumably included there due to behaviour and attitude, that could have been a wide demographic and choice of behaviour. By indicating feelings as a cause and symptom of madness the indignant and angry (see Perceval) were quickly judged as mad. Feelings, not bread or injustice, were therefore paramount in the construction of human personality. If Pinel does allude to injustice it is through the patient's reception, expressed as too much pride or vanity. Situation dominated all, in the sense of where they were then located. It is then judgement based on appearance. Although Pinel displaced medieval concepts of mental-illness, replacing both the supernatural and priests, he appears to have replaced it with the single point of clinical rationality and the clinician's voice. In effect, replacing one superstition with another. Moral archetypes, scarcely examined, predominated-such as avarice and pride, themselves complex emotion/ideas. At a time when hospitals were a mish-mash of small time criminals, battered wives, unwanted wives, parents and children Pinel judged it seems by situation not mental health problems. These may have become the 'personality disorder' candidates of later psychiatry. Renewing my research on this period it interested me that no official histories appear to make note of these activities, painting an unbelievably rosy picture of heroic doctors and humane treatments. Usually, they ignore or attempt to ignore the reality. It is historians who illuminate the truth.

So at this point we are I think caught up in ideas of place indicating mental instability, conditions solely identified by physicians, clinical authority and status constructing reality. How many such individuals Pinel treated is open to question-Pinel took a situational approach to madness, see above, if you were a patient in his hospital you were mentally ill after all. His assumption that everyone he met was mad or suffering from mental illness to some degree or another appears naïve. His attitude is no different from most doctors today, who see the world within a single cognitive dimension.

Certainly, from an early point in time morality and un-diagnosable mental orders were aligned, and the term anti-social becomes interchangeable with difference and unconventional. Foucault [72] rightly asserts that authority has replaced physical punishment, the absolute authority of physicians' ideas and experiences. Therefore, if Pinel chose to believe that all the people in Bicetre and Salpetrietre were mad, no matter what they told him about their reasons for being there, they were mad because he decided they were. The differences were largely, if you were in the asylum you were mad, if outside you were sane. This approach in addition connected failure, lack of employment with personality difficulties, problems rather than alternative lifestyles and individual choice. What will be seen is that those described by the medical profession as suffering from personality disorders appear to have no rationales-as cognition belongs to doctors only in doctor/patient relationships.

~~~~~~

[72]

tps://monoskop.org/images/1/14/Foucault_Michel_Madness_and_Civilization_A_History_of_Insanity_in_the_Age_of_Reason.pdf

Table 1

Description of DSM Personality Disorders

Personality disorder	Description
Paranoid	Pervasive pattern of distrust and suspiciousness of others
Schizoid	Pervasive pattern of detachment from social relationships; restricted range of emotional expression in interpersonal interactions
Schizotypal	Pervasive pattern of odd, eccentric behavior or thinking; perceptual distortions; discomfort in interpersonal interactions
Antisocial	Pervasive pattern of disregard for and violation of the rights of others
Borderline	Pervasive pattern of instability in interpersonal interactions, sense of self, and affect; marked impulsivity
Histrionic	Pervasive pattern of excessive yet shallow emotionality and attention-seeking
Narcissistic	Pervasive pattern of grandiosity, need for admiration, and lack of empathy
Avoidant	Pervasive pattern of inhibition and feelings of inadequacy in interpersonal interactions; hypersensitivity to negative evaluation
Dependent	Pervasive and excessive need to be taken care of; dependence on and submission to others
Obsessive-Compulsive	Pervasive pattern of preoccupation with orderliness, perfection, morality, and control

Each of the above is subject to rapid recalibration into day by day, and day to day, infractions that are simply part of general human nature. Taken by themselves they represent archetypes that accord to all of us in specific situations. The medical hook is the term 'pervasive', that is over-time, but such effects can be easily obtained through short-term or long-term situational episodes and experiences. The central problem here is the negative, at times sinister, interpretation in the DSM and elsewhere of common human traits.

4. Back to personality disorder again.

So now we have it. People can be mentally ill without actually being mentally ill, their illness consequent on the nature of both observer and observation. It is the observer, the doctor, who decides what is normal (sane) and abnormal (mentally ill). The clinical diagnoses now depends on subjectivity. We believe Pinel's diagnoses, even though they might have been simply of unfortunates, because of his authority and apparent understanding of mental illness. In such understanding resistance and anger become symptoms of mental illness. *'When a difficult patient has been assessed and treated fully without a favourable response, the problem is often reformulated as a diagnosis of primary personality disorder.'* (Tyrer et al: page 1) Remarks such as these can be successfully recalibrated as when a patient does not do as they are told (physician's authority) they will be judged as more ill than the original diagnosis or suffering from some form of illness because we cannot otherwise think of what to diagnose them. I have witnessed such behaviour myself from mental health professionals. The illness belongs thereby to the doctor, not the patient.

Going by Foucault's belief in Pinel's introduction of authoritarianism and absolutism,[73] in fact already there in the managers of private mental homes, the psychiatrist determined what a person suffered from and if someone was mad or not. They decided they had knowledge about others, which separated them from others. If you, the reader, went to see a psychiatrist they would decide what you suffer from, its nature, and you would have no say in the matter. Your possible insights, knowledge and intelligence would be snuffed out and in Foucault's language you would become the subject to the gaze, exploration of the physician. This does seem to be what occurs. From what clients have told me, you do not actually need to have problems. *Once a diagnosis is attached you become the diagnosis.* Also, anyone consulting a psychiatrist will later discover some category or another has been wilfully connected to them. That a doctor might have misunderstood something you said or did not properly hear you is not factored into any possible diagnosis-absolutism prevails.

Client's narrative: A break up with his girlfriend about to have his child involved my client going to court to get access. The ex-girlfriend made accusations about him which were followed through, and he was thereby held to be unstable. Ignoring the attitudes against him, knowing the courts and services would be biased, he thought only of his son. There was no evidence of mental instability but he came under observation. He was later told that if he had made the same accusations against his ex-partner there would have been less pressure on him. He told me he did not regret his choice of putting the child first, and as far as he was concerned he had done the right thing.

He met his son in a children's centre where his mental instability was a given. He was aware that his ex-partner was still telling stories about him so he refused to speak with her. That was seen as evidence of his mental instability. His ex-partner who had moved on into another relationship continued with her claims. My client told me that she was perceived as the rational one, a description my client laughed to scorn, and he thought, probably with justice, that she was manipulating them. He stated to me that he thought they believed themselves to have specialised knowledge and that they believed they knew the situation far better than they

---

73

tps://monoskop.org/images/1/14/Foucault_Michel_Madness_and_Civilization_A_History_of_Insanity_in_the_
Age_of_Reason.pdf (179)

actually did. The head therapist he described as extremely egotistic and arrogant (*Narcissistic Personality Disorder/Schizoid Personality Disorder*). At one point he was verbally abused by the staff, and he confided to his MP who knowing something of such matters stepped in.

Such stories give support to the behaviour of mental health professionals and their reconstructions of reality due to situational episodes and power. Their evidence for my client's instability was purely anecdotal and based on his gender; prejudice in effect. In addition, he felt the staff believed they had a right, indeed the authority, to treat people as they liked.

(This is a narrative therefore the ex-partner might have told it differently, and the staff in the reception centre, but it does not mean any were right as they all approached the matter with preconceptions and ideologies. The ideologies of psychiatrists impact on their judgements, and too much power given to any individual or group leads to abuse. In these situations, the professionals' view, whether it is right or wrong, dominates and excludes other points of view.)

Tyrer et al, itemises one apparently famous case or narrative in which a nobleman passing a peasant woman tossed her into a well, causing her death. Tyrer et al, are convinced that here we have a psychopath, but the problem, as they saw it, was the lack of evidence for a mental state-no hearing of voices or mood swings. The gentleman was imprisoned in the Bicetre under Pinel's care. Let us again look at a possible alternative or rather alternatives. Perhaps the peasant women had threatened him and his family at an earlier point, or he had experienced a seizure, a momentary condition of the mind, or it was an accident. As a nobleman during the French Revolution was all the evidence biased against him? We have a narrative according to Pinel and the authorities, not from the nobleman or unbiased witnesses- so we do not know what actually occurred.

Let us look again at another case, provided by an American doctor mentioned by Tryer et al, Benjamin Rush, the founder of American Psychiatry. A signer of The Declaration of Independence, Rush continued to use purging and bloodletting to extremes causing it is thought a large number of unnecessary deaths: he made mental patients in his care take mercury believing it was a cure-all: he ignored the results of his treatments, the bodies building up around him: he believed in coercion of mental patients and restraint, a form of Moral Treatment, forcing the doctors higher will onto others, and invented a restraint chair that to modern eyes looks like a form of torture. Was Rush insane or just a psychopath? Maybe he was just a fool or perhaps overwhelmed by his own power and others unwillingness to confront him. Alternative reality suggests that if he did not possess the power given to him by others he would and should have been incarcerated. He probably killed more people than famous mass-murderers. No one seems willing to suggest he was mad or subject to a personality disorder-but surely in the descriptions of such disorders he clearly was?

(Schizoid Personality Disorder, or perhaps suffering from Narcissistic Personality Disorder. In effect these are descriptions of a particular type-arrogant and conceited and careless about

the sufferings of others. But again, Rush demonstrated empathy on many occasions. The belief that certain human characteristics are 'disorders' is again situational. The same characteristics are not disorders if they are displayed by people in authority. Referencing Jung's collective unconscious, he did a great deal of good evidencing wisdom archetypes.)

The narratives of psychiatrists past and present would make up a book on suspected sufferers of personality disorder, but they had or have the power and apparent rationale to reject such a step. Dr William Sargant, famous in the 1960s, had an evangelical zeal for physical treatments of the mentally ill that might have shamed Benjamin Rush. He held that he could do whatever he liked with and to his patients in attempts to cure them of disorders he himself had diagnosed. He championed drug use on patients, often experimenting with new types of drugs, employed insulin shock therapy, used ECT freely and excessively no matter its effects and dangers. He famously wiped the memories of a 14 year old girl at the behest of her mother. Dogma preceded evidence.

From many standpoints he meets many of the criterion for personality disorder, but likely as not he diagnosed others with the complaint and permanently damaged them with his treatments. As a psychiatrist he was free to do so. (*Personality disorder recommended: Schizoid Personality Disorder. That is he found it difficult to properly relate to others. Considered by many to be autocratic he seemed unconcerned by the harm he did to others. Nevertheless so fluid are the DSM's terms that many others will do as well. It is worth noting that I have employed the same disorder for each professional therefore it appears all mental health professionals, their own reasoning goes, must suffer from Schizoid Personality Disorder/Anti-Social Personality Disorder. Referencing Jung's ideas once more, Sargant also wrote brilliant insightful books on psychology).*[74]

It seems that killing and harming others, if you are a doctor with a suitable rationale, placing you above the law and beyond psychiatric diagnosis, then your behaviour is fine, evidencing situation, power and status. The understanding conveyed by Tryer et al conveys both certainty and confusion. On page 464 the authors consider the fluidity of words in describing the nature of illnesses identified as mental illness but in fact not mental illness; an illness searching for complete taxonomy perhaps and hoping that different disciplines will accomplish the task? The medical profession needs a way indeed of describing social issues propounded mainly by individuals that require greater group clarity. At this stage it is and remains a debate over fitting language to psychiatric ambitions. Is Personality Disorder an illness or not, referencing Akiskal et al (1986), with many preferring borderline, but borderline to what? Extensive typologies are formed that may have less to do with scientific acuity than physician fantasy.

Abnormality of personality traits is one constant definition, but to what? Difficulties in social relationships (who does not?) and problems with perceptions (is that really a negative property?) As with previous attempts to understand this condition or conditions, it is done by psychiatry or psychiatrists without consultation with other experts within a narrow cultural context. Doctor's perceptions of the world alone constitute knowledge, a knowledge gained

---

[74]http://www.nickread.co.uk/articles/2010/03/visionary-or-disaster-a-perspective-on-william-sargant/ This website is written by Dr Read who described Sargant as 'dangerous'-a view of many of his peers who did nothing to stop him.

through Pinel's taxonomy, where all other people outside of the profession and strict forms of bourgeois behaviour determined by ideas of excess. The medical profession constructs beliefs on personality uncorroborated by other groups, that governments give them freedom to enforce.

5. Final Section:

This section will look at some of Pinel's case studies referencing Huneman's work; present day studies by working psychiatrists on personality disorder; and the DMS on personality disorder. Firstly, it has to be recognised that Pinel was an ideologue (Philippe Huneman) who believed certain things, such as analyses and confinement, and dogmatically stuck to them. I will demonstrate that the same is identifiable in the DSM.

Case B-

Both Case A and B in Huneman's short review are rooted in the violence of the Revolution and could be seen as moral, psychological and philosophical reactions to it. The Post Traumatic Stress Disorder, more worthy of its name as the emphasis is on cause not victim, which probably affected many early asylum inmates. While Pinel occasionally references the political environment of the time he does not appear to accord it possible causation in his young patient's illnesses.

Pinel's case histories have been considered at depth by Philippe Huneman but here only two will be referenced. Pinel's methods, as will be seen, are similar to present day case studies or papers on personality disorders which look at the disorder, consider doubts, pass over them and elaborate on the condition. Pinel's has an identifiable cause, usually contained within an event, with a causal relationship with madness contained within temporal anteriority.

Case B concerns a '*young religious enthusiast*' who arrives at the asylum after becoming overly affected by the abolition of the Catholic Church in France during the Revolution. According to Pinel his 'sombre misanthropy was without equal' as he focused perpetually on the torments of hell. He stopped eating. He rejected all comforts (which Pinel saw as clear evidence of his insanity). Pinel decided to resort to a ruse and instructed Pussin to go to his room and commanded a group of domestics to clang pots and pans, pretending to conduct him to hell. Soup was then put in his room and he was commanded to eat it under the threat of punishment if he did not. Caught between assured punishment in the temporal realm and possible torment in the hereafter, he ate the soup. He continued to eat and slept regularly and his health was gradually restored. His reason revived. Once he was back to some degree of reason he confessed to Pinel exactly how the ruse affected him.

Pinel presents the view of his own penetrating/supernatural vision, found also in Freud's case studies. He intuits the patient's inner thoughts and feelings and gives the impression that he knows the patient better than the patient knows himself. The internal conflict the patient undergoes is expertly managed by Pinel. Huneman decides that in fact, like many asylum owners of the day, such as Willis, he '*paradoxically induced, controlled, and fabricated*' the interior conflict. For both Willis and Pinel treatment was theatre. Huneman suggests that the hunger and thirst of the patient was directed by Pinel. According to Huneman, the intimacy of Pinel's approach requires an asylum-type environment (an environment controlled by the psychiatrist), which constructs the doctor/patient intimacy. He describes the final patient's confession is (apart from religious in nature) to Pinel evidence of the doctor's special gifts and the trust patients have in him, especially facing a tarrying experience orchestrated by the doctor.

Huneman considers how the case demonstrates the integration of any behaviour into paradigms of madness, once someone has been declared mad. So religious fervour is madness if the doctor has decided someone is mad, painting beautiful pictures can be related to madness if a doctor has declared someone mad, ambition, drives of any kind can be perceived in that fashion if a doctor has already declared that someone is mad. Case B decided to forgo luxury, therefore doing so, a reasonable position to take, was mad or irrational. Literary ambition, Case C, is madness, vainglory is madness-unless exhibited by the doctor. This story is like theatre, whereby everything occurs in the hospital, which is portrayed as a world of its own. By keeping the young man in the hospital, away from the outside world, and totally within Pinel's specific control a cure is affected.

In Case B we know nothing of events before the man arrived at the hospital. Was he brought or forced? To continue the theme above, not only was his religious fervour allied to madness but his Roman Catholicism as well. It is also possible that he was sent into the hospital for his own safety as he might have become a victim of fanatics or the state because of his loyalty to the Catholic Church. In fact the story of being tricked into sanity makes more sense if Case B realised he was in danger and decided to conform, that is go along with Pinel's ideas, pretend to be convinced by Pinel's reasoning and that way exhibit sanity. It seems clear that Pinel decided he was cured and perhaps a little later released him-perhaps suitably brainwashed.

Of equal importance is the young man's physical degeneration and revival as for Pinel this was essential in the journey to madness, where the body fails, and from madness to sanity where the body revives. The physical and mental for Pinel were inevitably linked.

Case C-The Friend.

A young man with a strong imagination comes to Paris to study. He believed he was destined to great things at the bar. Having assumed a vegetarian diet, which Pinel may have disapproved of, he secluded himself and spent hours at literary work. After a few months he was felled by violent migraines, frequent nose bleeds, oppression of the chest, bowel pains, flatulence, and over sensitivity. At first, Binel says he was happy, but often Pinel discovered him sunk in despair, asking Pinel to end his life. Pinel advised him to change his lifestyle, but his advice was rejected and the young man's problems increased. He then began to entreat Pinel to save his life. Pinel went walking with him but the fresh air failed to lift his spirits, and he began to go from mania to depression.

Huneman analyses the case, both Pinel's thinking and writing, which can be transposed onto his other cases.

The narrative demonstrates the patients need for the hospital and his emotional dependency on Pinel, and also of the special treatment offered there. Huneman[75] notes that the patient's escaping his attendant and only then committing suicide is a masked plea for patients to be permanently incarcerated, that is completely under the physician's control. Huneman points to Pidel's next paragraph in which he makes a case for the manager (Pinel) to have complete control of the asylum and the patients. One reason for this power is to deepen the intimacy with the patient-one that seems to have driven the patient in Case 2 to kill himself. Certainly Pinel claims that mental can illness can only be effectively treated in an asylum run by a governor/manager like him. In order for Pinel to control the young man, he needed the asylum as he could not do it anywhere else. Control and treatment, for Pinel, went hand in hand. As Huneman, when insisting on an 'autocratic manager' he is not insisting they have qualifications, only the personal authoritative mesmeric qualities he (like Willis) possessed. Pinel strongly identifies the hospital as the only place in which a cure can be effected. The hospital is present as the norm especially for the insane (3.3.2 page 21.) The hospital is the abode of the insane, the sane exist in the outside world.

Huneman[76] is perhaps being too kind to Pinel. The story can read several ways but one way is: Pinel meets a young man worn out by attempting literacy success. He has neglected himself. Pinel, possibly influenced by others related to the young man (see above) whom Pinel does not mention, takes the young man into the asylum-perhaps just for rest. While in there, Pinel does not leave him alone attempting that mental intimacy the young man may not want. The young man feels coerced and manipulated, and wants to escape but is prevented from doing so. Only when Pinel (hospital as norm) allows the young man outside the hospital does the young man find death-had he remained controlled and contained and not allowed outside, he might have survived. Pinel presents him as clutching a book of Plato's philosophy when he dies, indicating outside ideas have brought about his death. In fact, ancient Greek ideas (homosexuality?) as personified by Pythagoras and Plato, indeed any ideas other than Pinel's, have brought about his death, not Pinel's rational world of the hospital.

Pinel places himself at the centre of all his case studies, as does Freud, and the narrative pirouettes around his acuity.

Of importance here is Huneman's acceptance that Pinel within the controlled and contained environment of the hospital was reconstructing the meaning and nature of reality. Within it Pinel masters time or its perception (page 21). His case studies are in effect fiction-in terms of intentions, the growth of illness and its treatment. The modern day psychiatrist treats patients through the environment of his/her ideology, with taxonomy, whether of personality disorder or psychosis the prison in which and whereby patients can be controlled.

---

[75] Writing the case-Pinel as Psychiatrist. Institute of Histoire et de Philosophie des Sciences et des Techniques, CNRS/Universite Paris I Sorbonne.
[76] Writing the case-Pinel as Psychiatrist. Institute of Histoire et de Philosophie des Sciences et des Techniques, CNRS/Universite Paris I Sorbonne.

DSM-5: Diagnostic and Statistical Manual of Mental Disorders

The DSM contains generalisations, besides the mental state illnesses, that can be attributed to most people at some point or another and as can be seen I have employed some to describe the above psychiatrists in accordance with their behaviour, irrespective of the ideologies said to inform that behaviour. As has been noted, Personality Disorders are archetypal descriptions, which means they reference, and are designed as metaphors for shared behaviours. These do not represent individuals but are a continuation of Pinel's attempt to classify mental diseases as physical diseases were classified. They do not represent or need to represent individuals as they are thereby metaphors for shared group relationships. The individual is part of a greater whole with whom they apparently share behaviour or attitudes. Personality Disorders describe these existent or non-existent groups through elements of their behaviour or attitudes, but ignore those elements they do not share, concentrating on particular and peculiar aspects: the grumpy celebrity has a paranoid or schizoid personality disorder that requires treatment, except that no mention is made of his many friends and charitable work while the ideologically driven psychiatrist ticks all the accepted boxes of normality but kills people through overzealous treatments! Perhaps normality is the true myth here.

A

This paper, *Interpersonal Dysfunction in Personality Disorders: A Meta-Analytic Review,*[77] is taken from the DSM to add clarification to one seemingly free flowing disorder[78], written in a similarly fluid and strangely imprecise fashion. Such styles of writing are common in the papers attached to the DSM, reflecting its descriptive intentions.

The paper presents itself thus: *Personality disorders are defined in the current psychiatric diagnostic system as pervasive, inflexible, and stable patterns of thinking, feeling, behaving, and interacting with others.* Going on to admit that the very concept of personality disorder has been challenged, critics pointing out the descriptions ignore cultural differences, and have met that challenge with inclusion. Apart from this being a natural defence to reasonable, if it is or was a science why not before and does not such inclusions further testify to its cultural background, that is it is an expression of cultural phenomenon not recordable facets of human personality. The idea of personality as 'pervasive, inflexible, and stable patterns of thinking, feeling, behaving, and interacting is surely a phenomenon of most human beings, offset by education and varied experience. Commonly, these facets are found in religious societies en masse. Are all or a majority of people in these societies suffering an aligned personality disorder or is it just a phenomenon of human personality structured and organised through culture? Pinel himself had rigid thinking-thereby ideological-and by becoming psychiatrists, psychiatrists themselves contract to be part of fixed ideologies. Are all psychiatrists suffering from personality disorders?

---

[77]Sylia Wilson, Catherine B. Stroud, and C. Emily Durbin. NCBI. PMC. US National Library of Medicine. National Institute of Health.

[78] https://www.ncbi.nlm.nih.gov/pmc/articles/PMC5507693/

This indeed is the level that the discursive thinking revealed in the DSM is placed.

The gist of the paper is that personality disorder prevents people from getting on with others, although whether that is really to be considered an illness and its opposite (settling down in marriage with 2.5 children, steady employment with conflict) is to be embraced is surely a necessary matter of debate? Many people do not get on with others: greater intelligence, greater autonomy, greater talent or greater motivation and drive. The DSM, and constructs of personality order, deal only with negatives: it is puritanical, conventional, conforming thinking which seeks to establish a norm based on envy and castigate those who do not meet the norm. It meets Foucault's complaint against Pinel, page 197:

Very soon Pinel could write: "How necessary it is, in order to forestall hypochondria, melancholia, or mania, to follow the immutable laws of morality!"

The number of innovators, great artists, writers and scientists who meet definitions of personality disorder is considerable, not because they are mentally ill but because they sometimes break codes of morality (Rimbaud), or of lifestyle (Pessora) and they do so through intentionality-a property psychiatry denies the human objects it classifies.

Surely, this concerns social control, not illness?

As invariably with the DSM, which is to science what icecream is to icebergs, although what is not accepted in human behaviour, but is accepted (according to its compilers) is not accorded the slightest space, so although claiming scientific insight it does so in the vacuum of diagnostic empiricism, which in fact is no more than the compilation of mutually agreed anecdotes searching for an idea.

Further, the notion of fixed ideas, ie ideology, is the very method of understand psychiatry and its practitioners suffer from, based upon Pinel and fully demonstrated by the DSM. The term Pot, Kettle, Black comes immediately to mind.

64

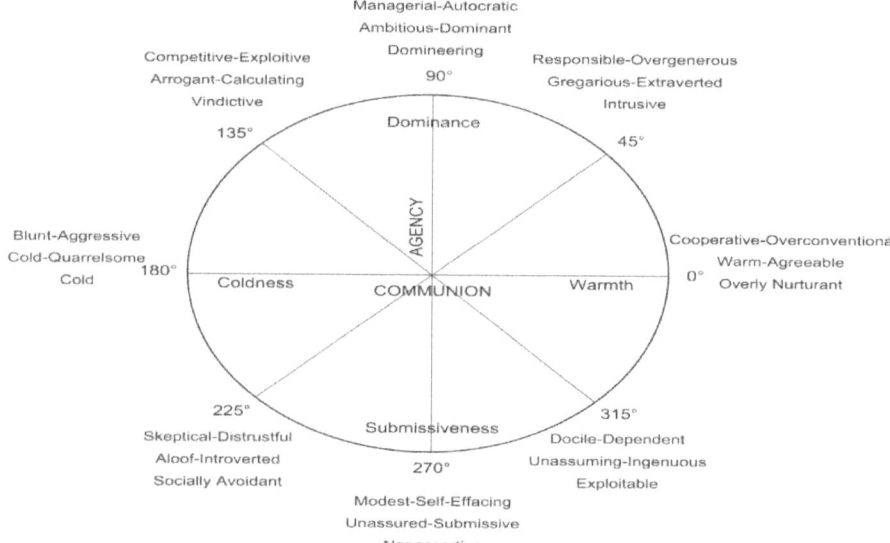

Graphs like these can be found in psychological papers, for example Myers-Briggs, an introspective self-report questionnaire. Or indeed in astrology. Psychiatry employs them for invasive, life changing treatments, reinforcing its authenticity, methodologies and status. In fact, I suggest they have little more genuine meaning than the results of visiting local clairvoyants and astrologers. The extremes of behaviour possible with each of the above can be dealt with outside of medical care (not all), and there is in fact no proof that medical care has any or much efficacy of cure in any of them. The above are little more than human characteristics pathologised, and their credibility depends solely on public gullibility.

B

The second paper in the DSM or from those elaborating on its descriptions:

The expansionist tendencies of psychiatry are perhaps most clearly exampled in the accompanying paper *Historical roots of histrionic personality disorder*[79] -that is people who vocalise feelings in a search for attention, find stress difficult and cannot deal with internal angst. The older term for this and for the majority of those now described as personality disorder was neurosis, but the more recent term has itself histrionic dimensions, attracts public attention and gives rose to physician intervention. Neurosis can be ignored but personality

[79] Filipa Novais, Andreia Araujo, Paula Godinho *Front Psychol*. 2015; 6: 1463. Published online 2015 Sep 25. doi: 10.3389/fpsyg.2015.01463

disorder, well that surely has to be deeply serious? The employment of *disorder* immediately raises the ante.

The authors link it to hysteria, which Freud placed in traumatic early experiences. The authors list a variety of disorders that emerged from hysteria, and the connection between Naming and archetypes becomes real as both employ (obviously) words to structure reality. Naming induces a reality. It is strange that the idea has been resurrected as its connection to patriarchal and misogynistic belief systems was long ago identified plus also the tendencies of male doctors to project onto female patients. Unfortunately psychiatry unlike psychoanalysis is not remotely thoughtful or aware of others' ideas. Freud's case involving a young female patient named Dora remains a warning for most psychotherapists of the therapist's own capacity for manipulation and being manipulated by men as well as women.

A psychotherapist knows that they can play a part in creating illness within a patient but psychiatrists have no understanding of their potential for an active role in the construction of illness. For Sargant, his destruction of brains was merely at best collateral damage pursuing a science. He played no part in causing illness within his patients. So psychiatrists feel their observational methods cannot possibly generate suspicion in patients, but note a patients' suspiciousness down as part of their paranoid personality disorder. Taking patient notes does not have to be accurate, but simply reflect the psychiatrist's diagnostic skills, which often consists of simply reading the DMS and memorising it.

Conclusion:

Psychiatry tends to radically misuse language. When for example it presents a Personality Disorder it is using language reframed and reformed for itself, constructed upon both its authority and ideology with both a clinical and popularising slant. Where Jung employs *complex*, psychiatry uses disorder implying confusion, conflict, social breakdown. It is presenting language as a tool of status and power over others not of clarification.

Taxonomies construct a reality. Instead of people with a number of clear differences, psychiatric taxonomies present people as groups and also fixed within that group, without individual identity, history or emotional processes. This takes us back to the earlier part of the last century: to sciences on racial differences, gender differences, eugenics and similar thinking; groups of individuals that seem the same because of shared characteristics, like skin colour. Taxonomies are a means of control: only white people can use this bus, rebellious people cannot be listened to, a politician or business person functions purely within the realm of their taxonomy-creating isolation and separation.

While Jung attempted to offset this problem by creating compilations of archetypes (taxonomies) within the individual and providing each individual with a past and future, psychiatry uses taxonomies to keep people in an eternal present-at the time of diagnosis-with an eternal, fixed identity represented by the diagnosis. It is in the end a means of tying patients/people to the medical profession in one form or another, the enforced intimacy and dependency that Huneman has noted.[80] The diagnosis stays on a patient's record until death

---

[80] Writing the case-Pinel as Psychiatrist. Institute of Histoire et de Philosophie des Sciences et des Techniques, CNRS/Universite Paris I Sorbonne.

and after and informs others, and the individual, of their identity. It is thereby a means for the mental health services to continually confirm their own group and individual authenticity.

The intellectual history of psychiatry.

This paper is the last but one in this short project, an addition to An Unusual Power, and looks at how psychiatrists developed their views, seeing their clients/patients as objects, relying on poor science, driven, I suggest by ideology not evidence based analysis. This paper describes the evolution of different strains of psychiatry-*Proprietor, Asylum, Dynamic,* and *Biological,* or as I have identified it, *Laboratory.* It will describe a professional group, often from the same demographic, driven by a search for status, defining itself through dogma and power, and expressing limited insight into the *human condition.* I will, apart from looking at and analysing the historical evidence, employ personal anecdotes, using client witness to treatments, and attempt to understand the significance of psychiatric case-studies, what they say about the profession, considering also an economic understanding of medicine and medical care. In the process, I will look at child prostitution in Victorian London, asylums in the UK and America, Freud, principal Victorian psychiatrists, *Proprietor, Asylum, Dynamic* and *Biological-Laboratory Psychiatry* and the economics related to psychiatric ideas and practices. This paper holds that the history of *Asylum Psychiatry,* the now dominant form, was and remains a search for legitimacy, not the history of a science.[81]

1. The Duel: Mind or Body.

Prior to the 1950s the pervasive understanding of mental illness was through psychoanalytical concepts of the unconscious, and covered a range of ideas and hypothesis. Freud and his followers dealt exclusively with those now suffering, according to psychiatry, personality disorders. Psychoanalysts did not deal usually with extreme cases such as psychosis. Nevertheless, where prevailing views were concerned, the ideas of psychoanalysis or closely allied to it dominated both the language and debate. Although many psychoanalysts were doctors, equally many were not [82]and represented the knowledgeable layperson of the kind the medical profession had struggled with for dominance in the past, deciding which ideology would in medical thinking.[83] The understanding of mental illness or health was constructed through psychotherapy, psychiatry, anthropology and other humanist disciplines. Different Cognitive Therapies emerged from '*talking therapies*' and in terms of quantitative surveys[84], are the most successful of all psychiatric interventions.[85]

---

[81] Scull. Madhouses, Mad-Doctors and Madmen: The Social History of Psychiatry in the Victorian era. Psychiatry in the Victorian era. Page 11. University of Pennsylvania Press. 1981.

[82] Delille, Emmanuel. Teaching the History of Psychiatry in the 1950s: Henri Ellenberger's Lectures at the Menninger Foundation. 2006 Varia. Zinbun No.47

[83] Much of the *Unusual Power* deals with this ideological struggle.

[84] https://www.ncbi.nlm.nih.gov/pmc/articles/PMC3742431/

[85] http://www.psychotherapyreferral.com/how-effective-is-cognitive-therapy.html

Psychiatry had taken a different and more sinister route, conducted behind closed doors with what has been called Asylum Psychiatry, considered differently to other forms.[86] This paper asserts that Asylum Psychiatry informs present-day psychiatry and provides the paradigms of the drugs and invasive treatments people are now likely to receive. This is psychiatry constructed around and upon the medical practitioner's views and experience of the world that can be seen in the ideas of Pinel[87] whereby the psychiatrist interprets and controls the patient's experience at the same time as effecting control over the patient. This is often done through pathologising processes.[88] Although Pinel is one of the originators of much *Asylum Psychiatry*, his concentration on the mind gives him a foot in both camps. Certainly his attempt (Emil Kraepelin: 1923) to marry philosophy and psychiatry would be foreign to most practicing psychiatrists.

The 19th century began with, in the UK and the USA, private hospitals managed by mad-doctors, proprietor-managers who professed and exhibited apparent knowledge of madness based on their possession of paying or paid for patients. Even though without systematic learning-many were either religious leaders (Tuke) or medical doctors-they claimed expertise and were deferred to.[89] This *mad-trade* established psychiatry's early links to business.[90] In the previous century patients, many not mad at all, were chained up, beaten and tortured as a method of getting rid of demons thought to lie behind their conditions or as with Hogarth's *The Rake's Progress* punishment for the libertine lifestyle. The move to Moral Treatment[91], humanitarian care as a method of cure, was based on competition between private mad houses as well as the Enlightenment. In France mad-houses were early aligned to the state while in the UK doctors in general became politicised (enounced in power) as the result of concepts of the masses and the political influence of the masses, combined with ideas of the political importance of health. By 1848 there were 148 private mad-houses in the UK plying a decent trade, branding themselves by the nature of their accommodation, its location, care of inmates and the persuasive power of their ideologies, but after that date the numbers began to fall as the result of competition with the new county asylums.[92]

Competition over treatments:

Extensive use was m ade of the "Tranquilizer" introduced by Rush. This restraining chair was equipped with sup- ports to which the body, legs, and arms could be lashed. In a few hours, according to Willis, it would make the most stubborn and irrascible patient gentle and submis-

---

[86] An Unusual Power: Madhouses: Sane or Insane?https://www.researchgate.net/publication/320173717_An_Unusual_Power_Madhouses_Sane_or_Insane

[87] Ed. Bynum, Porter, Shepherd. *Introduction*.The Anatomy of Madness. Essays in the History of Psychiatry. Vol III. The Asylum and its Psychiatry. Routledge. Taylor and Francis Group. London and New York.

[88] Foucault, Michel. Madness and Civilisation.

[89] Parry-Jones, William L. The Trade in Lunacy. Routledge 2013.

[90] Parry-Jones, William L. The Trade in Lunacy. Routledge 2013.

[91] https://psychologydictionary.org/moral-treatment/ This description is succinct, but for a deeper view An Unusual Power: Madhouses: Sane or Insane?https://www.researchgate.net/publication/320173717_An_Unusual_Power_Madhouses_Sane_or_Insane

[92] Parry-Jones, William L. English private madhouses in the eighteenth and nineteenth centuries. Proc R Soc Med. 1973 Jul; 66(7): 659–664.

sive. Horn remarked that it had a remarkable effect on the psychology of the patient "He must tolerate having his body in an uncomfortable or a painful position . . . The new and unpleasant situation engages his attention and directs it toward something external. Sooner or later he regains his self-esteem. He often emerges calm, thought- ful and tractable. " Groos treasured the restraining chair to such an extent that he repeatedly stated, according to Roller, that without it he would not care to be an alienist. Heinroth publicly recommended it as the best restraining device known to him for transforming many unruly individuals in dark, isolated places into gentle, submissive men and women. Jacobi took issue with him and cited a patient who had spent six consecutive months in the re- straining chair. Blumroder also maintained that restraint aggravated the lunatic's condition, prolonging and in- tensifying his resistance. "The sanest man would soon agree with me," he added, "if he spent half an hour on a restraining chair, unable to scratch a fleabite."

Emil Kraepelin. One Hundred Years of Psychiatry. Originally published c 1923.[93]

The competition between private mad-houses was played out through the application and efficacy of Moral Treatment, with unsubstantiated claims made, a common trait in psychiatry, alongside a belief in a connection between moral virtue and sanity, the proprietor or Superintendent's Will-Francis Willis and Pinel-and patients' absorption of the Mad-House Superintendent's ideology. Foucault[94] was correct in dismissing this as controlling through moral concepts of normality. Pinel's case studies, which show him as central, a man of mesmeric personality and considerable perspicuity demonstrate this-especially given his insistence for closed asylums in which the Superintendent/Alienist decides everything. [95]

Nevertheless, economics has remained at the heart of mental health care and constitutes a hidden driver of its ideologies.

The desire for professional and social status is visible in Pinel, Benjamin Rush, Tuke and, Francis Willis, the bullying alienist for George III, which provides one reason why they intellectualised their activities, and why this drive remained within the Asylum mad-doctors until their evolution into psychiatrists, relaxing only with the profession's attainment as the dominant ideology in mental health from the 1950s. From the time of Pinel, et al, they sought a science that would prove convincing. [96] This was a profession that often treated the occupants of their facilities badly, creating thereby a poor image for themselves. Although it is possible to justify Asylum-Psychiatry abuses, its extent and continuance is another matter, involving alteration of perception in both doctor and patient, the asylum a place of different constructed realities to the world beyond its doors.

Pinel popularised the need to make observations of patients and take notes, in that way building up data, which often reflected his interest in philosophy. This process became extensively

---

[93] https://archive.org/stream/onehundredyearso011002mbp/onehundredyearso011002mbp_djvu.txt
[94] Madness and Civilisation.
[95] Huneman, Philippe. Writing the case-Pinel as Psychiatrist. Institute of Histoire et de Philosophie des Sciences et des Techniques, CNRS/Universite Paris I Sorbonne.
[96] An Unusual Power: Madhouses: Sane or Insane?https://www.researchgate.net/publication/320173717_An_Unusual_Power_Madhouses_Sane_or_Insane

employed adding to the use of descriptive text in assessing patients. This is considered an early scientific method but equally is open to mistakes and misunderstandings. It provides anecdotes and the notion that people can be categorised into groups.

The drive for status has affected the profession's development [97] as has the role of Superintendents of mad-houses; alienists and psychiatrists (a term popularised by the end of the 19th century) constructing controlling behaviour as well as many present psychiatric ideas within the closed societies they ruled over. The arrival of asylums gave alienists the chance to develop theories, which evolved into Moral Treatment, and from there moral psychiatry where normality became confused with moral correctness. Of significance is that alienists/medical Superintendents were left alone and accorded specialist status early on, and within the asylums allowed to do whatever they wished. Mental health remained a mystery, with supernatural overtures, unravelled by magicians. Moral Treatment was the first of many doubtful ideas that have continued up to the present day based on dubious ideologies that masqueraded and masquerade as science. From the beginning notions of control pervaded treatments, with hypothesis tested out by force. Philippe Pinel in his Memoirs on Madness (1794), a political document that made a play for his own increased status, claimed that psychiatry needed to *'dominate agitated madmen while respecting human rights.'*[98] By and large, psychiatry has respected the first and ignored the second assertion.

Below are the factors that developed throughout the 19th century:[99]

1. Left alone by outside authorities, developing their own ideas and cures without engaging in debate with other groups.
2. Claiming specialist knowledge and framing that knowledge in several ways usually without recourse to scientific testing.
3. Convincing others of the efficacy of their treatments and ideas, no matter how fanciful.
4. Driven by a need for professional and personal status
5. Seeking scientific explanation and conversely a suitable scientific ideology
6. The compulsion to control
7. Each of these informed the profession's need to embrace and enact all kinds of treatment.
8. Established in psychiatry the original observer function of physician from the Renaissance. The observer role was re-constructed as scientific and has been used since.
9. The belief that patients are not negatively affected by their treatments, many of which resembled torture.
10. The belief that the entire world is mentally ill, or potentially so, but by some extremely odd chance not themselves.

[97] Pinel, Philippe. Memoirs on Madness.
[98] https://ajp.psychiatryonline.org/doi/abs/10.1176/ajp.149.6.725
[99] Scull, Mackenzie, Hervey: Masters of Bedlam: The Transformation of the Mad-Doctors' Trade. Princeton University Press. 1996.

The population of asylums grew by well over 100% by the end of the century.[100] That can be understood through increases in the world population, the ideological and psychological problems associated with capitalist societies where working is by itself a measure of normality, and with corresponding time pressures. It may again be due to statement No.10.

When private mental hospitals or care homes were established they would have brought additional money and work into an area, increased production of local foodstuffs and generally stimulated a local economy. When county asylums were established this general process was accentuated. In addition, as noted, professions were created-psychiatrists, mental health nurses, and, in time, social workers, welfare workers, who also stimulated by their presence local economies and general education. These benefits required an increasing number of patients, and the more people who were judged mentally ill the greater was the general economic impact. The increased number of mentally ill being cared for in Asylums might also have been the result of Alienists' desire for status, attention and acclaim. The more people diagnosed as mentally ill the more influential the profession became. A similar economic/status set of paradigms is encouraging the expansion of mentally-ill tropes today.

Status, then science.

Henry Maudsley for example was an upwardly mobile gentleman who achieved high social status, although originally a humble Asylum Superintendent, and wrote in *Pathology of Mind* (chap. *The Causation and Prevention of Insanity*)[101] a series of descriptive vignettes about people of lower social status and their decent into grumbling discontent presented as insanity. [102]He was one of several celebrity alienists. His writings display literary flourish but seem also a template for the DSM, descriptive evocations of type with little genuine science, no exploration of environment, and analysis based on social and intellectual superiority. It is both observational and anecdotal. Science, true science, should perhaps not display attitude. His notion of madness (page 261) flits between gloominess and loss of control, symbolised by rampaging animals, labelling epilepsy as a human form of the disease. He nevertheless, set up his hospital, named after him, with recovery as its main aim. This is in contrast to modern psychiatry which holds on to mental health patients until death (if it can) and succeeds in often doing so through persistent medication (This will be dealt with later).

2. Construction of ideas.

In the early part of the 19th century several views were considered as the reason for madness; sin (Heinroth: page 32), uncontrolled passions (Ideler: page 37), a number of others began to assert that insanity had physical origins. The separation between mind and body with one paradigm dominating and then another, seems ideologically backward, and yet it continues. Guislain (Kraepelin: 46) associated suicide with inflammation of the intestines (in line with a recent paper I read, believe it or not, suggesting something of the same-stomach bugs cause depression, modified, of course by drugs). Muller and Vering (124) held that reading books too

---

[100] An Anatomy of Madness. Vol. III Introduction.
[101] 3rd edition. D. Appleton and Company. New York. 1880.
[102] MacMillan and Co. 1879.

fast caused women to go mad, but then Willis put insanity amongst young men down to too much study (Kraepelin:49- they certainly clearly had a low opinion of women and scholarly youths).

According to Sonnenstein's system, disobedience and bad conduct ought to be punished severely. w Punishment ought to be meted out as speedily as possible following an investigation of the offense." Reil stated that since the in- sane were devoid of inner motivation, they had to be com- pelled to allow themselves to be influenced from without. He explained that the insane had to be trained in the same way as animals and children: "Rewards that bring pleas- ure and punishments that bring displeasure should be meted out in a proportion calculated to lead patients back to the path which is necessary and proper for them and which will cause them to be submissive and to practice strict obedience. He thought that people who misbehaved or were deceitful, malicious, disobedient or recalcitrant, and who at the same time were cognizant of their misconduct and of the purpose of the punishment to which they were being subjected, could be helped by corrective training. They ought, however, to be punished only at the direction of the superintendent and by a designated official; switches of bullwhips should be used, but never inordinately and cruelly or in a manner injurious to the health; punishment should never be meted out during an emotional outburst and should always be effected in the presence on others. Similarly, he reasoned that isolation, hunger, and defama- tion were important corrective measures. Conversely, patients ought to have their attention called to paragons of virtue drawn from ancient and modern history and to episodes in their own lives; where feasible, they should

Emil Kraepelin: page 77. One Hundred Years of Psychiatry. Originally published c 1923.[103]

Kraepelin wrote about these interesting psychiatric judgements in order to demonstrate that his science, compared to Moral Treatments and Philosophy, was infinitely better, although of course science is a philosophy dependent on validation through agreed methods of examination. Kraepelin (124) is commonly regarded as the first true psychiatrist, that is he declared that madness is a disease of the brain and advocated research on animals, whose brains although smaller than ours with many different properties are after all brains too. He advocated keeping patients under constant surveillance (124), like lab rats. In this kind of thinking we have the roots of *Laboratory Psychiatry*. Kraepelin was more astute than that although his work takes too much from the effects of syphilis on the brain as a guide to other forms of madness, and perhaps he would have been shocked by the intellectual trough of present-day psychiatric thinking with its myopic concern with drugs alongside the delusional conviction of their efficacy and harmless nature.

Asylum Psychiatry was formed within hospitals and reflects (Scull, Mackenzie, Hervey: 1996) the control methods and management tendencies of its development. Asylum Psychiatry sees the whole world as its subject-matter, as one universal hospital, providing another explanation perhaps for the profession´s expansion and the current obsession with mental health. Throughout the 19th century psychiatry developed, without at any point reflecting scientific

---

[103] https://archive.org/stream/onehundredyearso011002mbp/onehundredyearso011002mbp_djvu.txt

mores, moving from Asylum or hospital psychiatry to office psychiatry (out-patient), physical psychiatry (ECT and Lobotomy-although offshoots of *Asylum Psychiatry* where lethal or dangerous practices were not uncommon) and from there to *Laboratory* or *Biological Psychiatry*. Throughout this time it constructed categorising, based on descriptive processes (demonstrated by Henry Maudsley above), invasive treatments where the body was and is perceived as an extension of the troubled mind and also a pathway for cures, resembling the earlier processes of exorcism. If the body is tortured sufficiently the insanity will retreat. Like the poor and mad the body was viewed as an object: a passive receptacle for ECT, coma induced therapy, and drug therapy-shocking, beating and injecting. This paper holds that psychiatric treatments were required to be obvious, visible and recordable.[104] They were often theatre, a way of proving physician efficacy and also of simply demonstrating that something was being done.

Language becomes confused; pathologising exchange.

This paper will consider how ideas of mental health and its cures changed in the second half of the last century, becoming based even less on genuine science. From this form we will trace its evolution in *Laboratory Psychiatry*, in which it still plays a vigorous part although not as solidly reductionist as the latter. Nor must it be seen, as Foucault does (1965), as largely harmful, as for many it gave a quality of life they may not otherwise have known, a relative oasis in a very harsh world. For that, they would have perhaps been happy to compromise their dignity and autonomy, to be seen as, at various times, childish, or for some animal like (Maudsley: 1880: 261), violent, finding themselves in a world of *observation and judgement* (Foucault: 1965)[105] where their actions were filled with pathological meaning (Michel Foucault: *Madness and Civilisation*. 1965)[106], every gesture and grimace confirming madness.

We certainly now see the interactive mannerisms of the psychiatrist emerge, where madness, as first encountered in the asylum, is all-inclusive. Everything about the mad person-subjected to *observation and judgement*-is representative of madness: drawing a picture, working out a maths problem, reading the same book more than once, loving flowers, loving people, enjoying comedies on TV, police narratives or horror. Once the psychiatrist's processes of *observation and judgement* have come into play, there is no escape for the patient. They are caught up in a prison of prejudice (mental health professionals often stigmatise more than those outside of the profession, holding fixed ideas about those judged mentally ill), where reason has failed. The psychiatrist's *observation and judgement* becomes un-reason or madness-it becomes paranoiac projection, subjecting language to the processes of pathologising.

As:

a) *Managerial-Autocratic/Ambitious-Dominant=Domineering*
b) *Responsible-Overgenerous/Gregarious-Extraverted=Intrusive*

---

[104] An Unusual Power: Sane or Insane.
[105] https://monoskop.org/images/1/14/Foucault_Michel_Madness_and_Civilization_A_History_of_Insanity_in_the_Age_of_Reason.pdf
[106] https://monoskop.org/images/1/14/Foucault_Michel_Madness_and_Civilization_A_History_of_Insanity_in_the_Age_of_Reason.pdf

c) *Docile-Dependent/Unassuming-Ingenuous=Exploitable* (DSM)

Madness and personality disorder or psychiatric projection? A) A creative business entrepreneur B) A charity worker C) Quiet and kindly.

And: Depress-I am depressed=unhappy, sad, a temporary state

Becomes Depression-changing an adjective into a noun.

I am or feel unhappy suffers the same semantic alteration. As does also *I am anxious.*

I am vulnerable through the process of *observation and judgement* becomes I suffer from personality disorder, in that both language and content are changed. The psychiatrist's very *judgement* reshapes reality.

Behaviour assumes semantic and value content. In Victorian times, politeness, good manners, sociability and conformity were now the attributes of sanity, and the reverse obviously that of the mad. (Scull, Mackenzie, Hervey: 1996). Even more, members of mental health services still regard rebellion as mental instability. Introspection, the ability to be by yourself was another indication (Scull, Mackenzie, Hervey: 1996). Clearly, the template for sanity, according to *Madhouses, Mad-Doctors and Madmen. The Social History of Psychiatry in the Victorian Period* (Scull, Mackenzie, Hervey: 1996) quoting important psychiatrists of the time-Maudsley, Clouston, Bevan Lewis, Savage, Blandford and Craig-was gregariousness, employment and no doubt a long term marriage. Of course sex, drugs and enjoying life brought on madness.

While hilarity at such poor ideas and thinking is justified, what if modern psychiatrists are actually no better as is indicated above? In fact, the relationship between the alienist and patient fits into the master/servant dichotomy of the time, with the belief in superiority of class prevalent then and later. The asylum became the manor house, its frontage exploiting the connection. The alienists had merely internalised common cultural perceptions. The psychiatrist's *judgement* is invested with illusions of professional expertise.

Forcible Re-Socialisation:

Anatomy of Madness Vol. III, 1996, points also to an abandonment of individual treatments, and the forcible re-socialisation of the mad, to get them away from self-absorption, a point actually made by Freud and still common in psychiatric thinking. Anatomy of Madness Vol. III references the categorisation of irritable nervous children, and how not to stimulate them (Henry Maudsley: Chap. *The Insanity of Early Life: 1879*). These ideas again seem common to community-based understandings of behaviour, of fitting in to the group, in other words express paradigms of conformity. Another belief in the development of madness and its production of introspection and morbidity was masturbation, a Victorian obsession.

Many years ago I came across some remarkably heavy well-preserved tomes detailing case studies based on masturbation as the central cause of morbidity, and, perhaps because no one took the descriptions so seriously then (although some psychiatrists still did), I saw them as the professional's fantasy. In Victorian times masturbation apparently lead teenage boys into the torments of psychosis. According to Thomas Clouston, a renowned Scottish psychiatrist, (*An Anatomy of Madness:Vol:III*, page 88) masturbation could lead to religiosity and intense morbidity, but, as usual with Asylum Psychiatry, shows no connection to family or environment. Bevan Lewis (*Academy of Madness: Vol. III* page 88 [107]) another eminent psychiatrist of the time, talked of the '*morbid subjectivity*' of the habitual masturbator and writes of the '*narrow, repulsive egotism*' of sufferers inserting a subjectivity into his arguments, common then and now, although heavily disguised.

The concentration on masturbation with connotations of '*filth*' and '*guilt*' were projected onto the mad, but this is even stranger given the commonplace nature of prostitution as a consequence of poverty, which many eminent psychiatrists may have taken advantage of, as well as engaging in child prostitution of both boys and girls. [108] Certainly, both were very visible. We actually know very little about the inner life of the celebrated Asylum Superintendents, their sexual inclinations and general behaviour, which like their hospitals were closed books. We know that Upper Middle Class professionals were known to take advantage of the East End poor, as seen in memoirs and life-stories (Oscar Wilde and his lover Bosie). The medical obsession with masturbation, whatever its rationale (largely Abrahamic) may therefore have belonged mainly to that class and not the poor, who like the mad were seen as the Other, objects to be exploited.

Paedophilia was not then seen as a mental illness as it is now, one of the personality disorders that although unpleasant cannot be properly dealt with by placing it into the psychiatric realm where the most recent claim is that, of course, it can be treated with drugs. I dealt with this in one of the previous papers pointing out that the proposed remedy is no more than drug induced castration no matter the scientific claims for the proposed treatment. One possible reason for its exclusion in Victorian times is that many medical men may have utilised the available '*trade*' themselves and therefore considered it normal. Many prominent men did, so the possibility is real enough. In much of Victorian society the poor were not important and were there for well-to-do men's pleasure or distraction.

The masturbation hypothesis lead me to consider then, many years ago, if other psychiatric beliefs were fantasy based on the construction of alternative worlds in the self-referencing, abnormal environments of asylums where the doctor was king, even god, that many of their ideas were and are not properly tested but exist in a liminal world controlled by mental health professionals in which alternative realities are dismissed. The hypothesis of Victorian gentlemen tend to be viewed simply as ideas, no matter if wrong, without a day to day context and genesis in their own lives. There are perceivable reasons for this: their middle class status during a time when occupying such a class gave an individual certain attributes as well as a specific psychology gleaned from high status and property owning with its Lockean perceptions of citizenship, individuality and possession; the illusion that they were concerned with science; the fact that their ideas were mainly constructed in the self-referencing environment of the asylum and not the greater world.

Psychiatric case studies will again be examined here in order to unravel psychiatric minds and systems of proof, to analyse how they convince and whether their ideas are actually true. Each, I have found fit a similar format. Moral judgements of character have been exchanged for constructs of abnormality, moral significance given to morality (page 89). Madness has

---

[107] Textbook of Mental Diseases. Charles Griffen &Co. 1889. Page 354.
[108] Mayhew, Henry. *The Longer Underworld in the Victorian Period: Authentic first person accounts by beggars, thieves and prostitutes.* 1862. Ebook by various suppliers.

replaced good and bad, corrupt and pure (normality is pure). Foucault (1965) argued similarly about the Moral Treatments of Pinel but such views continued and again remain-one need only to read the recent, as well as previous, DSM. My recent paper *A follow-on from Dangers of Psychotropic Drugs: A consideration of the Monoamine Hypothesis* examines the continued connection between morality and diagnosis within psychiatry.

It is easy to misunderstand the Victorian's delineations of mental illness, for the same tendencies exist now. Descriptive phrasing is masquerading as clinical judgement. Insanity can carry the meaning of loss of control and not represent scientific judgement: domineering can mean an annoying characteristic but also indicate insanity, see above. There is often little clarity of thinking. Psychiatry perceives its members as being normal, that is superior to mental health sufferers, more in touch with the rational world-they have work, money and power after all. Although much experimental work has been done in the effects of observation, demonstrating how it alters the behaviour of those being observed, the message has not reached society because of their reluctance to consider ideas from other disciplines. The rules of observation common to modern psychology[109] would have been unknown to Kraepelin and his contemporaries. The alteration of perception that occurs would be unknown to most psychiatric workers today, as would the unscientific nature of their actions.

Christine Stevenson (*Madness and the Picturesque in the Kingdom of Denmark: Anatomy of Madness Vol. III* Chapter 1) records the appearance also of a relatively new phenomenon: the belief that the number of mad people in the world was far more than in the various asylums, that the world was full of the mad in the same or a similar way people would later declare that Communists had infiltrated American society or space-aliens were amongst us disguised as lizards (page 108). I have noticed this with many mental health workers I have spoken to in work and in my travels. To impress this point on a personal level, a mental health nurse of my acquaintance would ask every new friend or boyfriend if they were mad, convinced that everyone around her was or was likely to be. She had been brought up in an asylum where the father worked as a superintendent, and upon adulthood had trained in the profession-therefore like many psychiatrists that is all she knew.

Enrico Morselli, a celebrated Italian psychiatrist, claimed that the number of 'mad' people was in fact far, far more than anyone imagined, and they escaped hospitalisation and '*official controls and consideration*', predicting Foucault's understanding. Psychiatrists routinely express this conviction; that the undiscovered mad need to be taken care of for their own sake. These convictions fill the pages of the DSM where any individuality is re-constituted as a form of mental illness (see above). Those who do not conform, the list in the DSM is long, need psychiatric care, the failed, the lazy (work being one measure of normality) the impolite, bad-mannered, nasty, creative-all clearly suffering from mental illness as subjected to psychiatric *observation and judgement*. Attached to each thoroughly normal (sic) description the DSM compilers attach 'excess' as the accompanying process towards pathologising. Henry Maudsley had taught Morselli that people were infinitely variable, not replete with talent, intellectual differences, some humorous, some dull, but in fact various in real or potential madness. Everyone was, and is mad, except by chance for them.

---

[109] https://www.simplypsychology.org/observation.html

Again, the more extreme obsessions may be of the time and may reflect the fear of invasion that gripped European nations at the end of the Victorian period. Britain feared invasion from France and then Germany, for example. H. G. Wells War of the Worlds also expressed these common anxieties.

Psychiatry and science:

The evolution from alienist to psychiatrist was one of status and respectability within the processes of management and ideology. Part of the process was to attach their profession to science. Hospitals had been set up, certainly by Pinel and others, as places where patients could be studied (experimented on) and cures could be effected[110]. For all the dubious claims of asylums and the appalling things that went on in them the editors (Scull, Mackenzie, Hervey: 1996) remind us that things were worse for those clearly deranged (I will leave the description for the moment). By the end of the century it was clear that they were not going to be successful at effecting cures. In fact, they were caught perhaps between a managerial role, the true role of psychiatrists until recently, and exhibiting medical expertise as mind doctors-curing psychiatric disease in the same way surgeons and ordinary family doctors occasionally cured. They perhaps needed dramatic therapies, creating the medical theatre that attracted attention and distracted from failure. This as will soon be seen is one rationale behind drug therapies, the much sought after cures that provided valediction for the profession. It also provides the rationale for the professions desire for control of others, and for never letting people go.

Asylums were built according to the separation of roles, with staff occupying one section separated according to class as determined by job roles, the doctors placed at a distance from the care staff, with patients housed in another part of the building according to diagnosis. They were self-contained worlds where patients were separated from outside world, had no autonomy with their identity and *Self* determined by various members of staff. Diagnosis became identity, as it remained in the next century, and, in fact, as it remains now. DSM provides identity through naming and classifying, the real person disappearing before and behind psychiatric gaze. Later, spirituality was discouraged as a root of madness, and, in fact, a madness itself.[111] Art was purely therapeutic and artistic drive denied. Becoming an exemplary patient was possible but not a great runner, writer, academic or even an average one. An excess, even of achievement, was deemed insanity. The DSM, an extension of *Asylum Psychiatry*, is a way to identify and separate people, owing its format to divisions of colour in slave-based America, Phrenology and Astrology.

Psychiatry was early associated with control, seen within Pinel's, and other early proprietors like Willis, thinking, and also with false imprisonment. In the USA, after the Civil War there was discussion amongst asylum Superintendents to have people committed by force, without

---

[110] Bynum, Porter, Shepherd. The Anatomy of Madness. Essays in the History of Psychiatry. Vol. 111. The Asylum and its Psychiatry. Routledge. 2004.

[111]Bynum, Porter, Shepherd. The Anatomy of Madness. Essays in the History of Psychiatry. Vol. 111. The Asylum and its Psychiatry. Routledge. 2004.

consent, through the law, but this was foiled by a recent, notorious case of a Mrs Packward, a fighter for women's rights, imprisoned by her husband in an asylum for three years because of theological disagreements with him. Freed, and back at home, her husband imprisoned her in the house and tried to have her committed again. The Superintendents´ request for the said law failed accordingly, judged dangerous by the courts as the result of their own dubious standards.[112]

The Packward case is interesting because the same procedures are likely now, in some ways, as then. Drugs are now the preferred method of silencing up argumentative relatives although a law passed by Tony Blair in the UK before his welcome departure from politics actually guaranteed the very same. In 1777 the Madhouses Act was passed through the British parliament to deal with the same problem with Madhouses being used as private prisons for unwanted relatives-a role served by psychiatry since. At that time in the USA, although not long ago, husbands too had the right by law to commit their wives to asylums. According to her religious husband, she had grown uppity, arguing with him. This to him was evidence of madness. He arranged for a doctor to visit her incognito, who, upon hearing her complaints against her husband too decided she was insane. Out of the blue, a few days later, she was committed. For the next three years bevies of psychiatrists treating her tried to convince her she was mad. In a catch-22 situation, once she admitted she was insane she would be on the way back to sanity. Eventually she was released, after pressure from her children, as incurable. A diagnosis that depended on her refusing to admit she was mad in the first place. After more battles with her husband in court, with a number of neighbours called who testified on her behalf, she was exonerated-the case was summed up by another doctor who asserted (1867): 'I do not declare people mad because their views differ from mine.'

In Victorian times, lack of acquiescence to a psychiatrist made you incurably mad, as it still does. Some historians of the period and most psychiatrists deny false imprisonment, but that claimants were anyway mentally ill but the claims follow the same or similar patterns. Those incarcerated were victims already of domineering personalities, or they had been judged of an immoral disposition-therefore mad. Scull[113]deals with the matter by pointing to the value-laden diagnosis of psychiatrists then (and now). No psychiatric diagnosis is ever free of some set of values.

4. Where it arrived.

Psychiatric concepts have tended to on the one hand insist on primacy and on the other hand lack the complexity of other viewpoints. As a group, it tends thereby to take the view that there is only one view, and that is ours.

In the 19th century, depression was seen as melancholy that is the other side of mania. The version today is revamped, more about fashion than actuality. Pinel of course envisioned depression as the result of an inability to reach desires along with moral faults, too much desire for single things, coupled with hubris. Diagnosed elsewhere depression was seen as reduced

---

[112] https://www.nlm.nih.gov/hmd/diseases/debates.html

[113] Madhouses, Mad-Doctors and Madmen: The Social History of Psychiatry in the Victorian era. University of Pennsylvania Press. 1981.

output, less interest or less energy.[114] From this period too we get descriptive ideas of mental complaints, expressed as diseases that affect sufferers in the same fashion and in the same way against intuitive concepts of normality. Pinel saw his clients as ideally expressing illness within the hospital and the outside world as having, in some of the most deadly periods in France, no effect on people's minds while at the same time likely to corrupt his patients if they re-entered it.

Compared to Pinel who endeavoured to develop psychiatric concepts to create status and further his career, the American psychiatrist Ray seems more concerned to establish its parameters through his *Treatise on the Medical Jurisprudence of Insanity*.[115] In my *Unusual Power* papers prior to this study of psychiatry, I have noted how important jurisdiction had been from medieval times in establishing concepts of madness-the inability to handle everyday affairs, especially to do with property transactions, was one. Likewise it has been touched on here in the 1867 court judgement on physician's powers above and the previous judgement in Britain on the kidnapping and imprisoning of wives on the word of disappointed or greedy husbands. These activities nevertheless continued. Psychiatrists had constructed their own world, and within it they were the law. Their perceptions ruled and overruled. [116]

Architecture:

Hospital architecture, location and layout were considered in depth.[117] The hospital was considered part of the patients' cure. Peter Cracknell completed research into American asylums, many of which appeared elsewhere, in 2004. He reported five different designs: Radial, with wards radiating out from a central core like a prison: Corridor plan, with the administration in the centre and wards flanking it: Pavilion Plan, with long linear corridor extending either side of an administration block: Dual Pavilion, consisting of administration and service blocks flanked by long corridors which were flanked by wards: Radial Pavilion, semi-circular services block with wards radiating out: Echelon Plan, which superseded the Pavilion Plans in 1880: Colony Plan, with blocks dispersed.

Most asylums were constructed to allow easy observation of patients. Layout of hospitals further encouraged the categorisation of patients, culturally fixing certain constructs to do with mental illness. The designs above centred everything upon staff, the running of the hospital, with patients away from the centre.

At this distant point we cannot know whether the patients should have been there or if the reasons were correct. These were insular environments cutting the inhabitants off from the outside world. but the notion of mental illness, albeit its tendency to respond favourably to domineering parents or spouses (something that remains whenever victims are not protected) was much narrower and depended on a recognisable inability for some people to exist normally. Nevertheless, it must be asked how much of psychiatrists' actions created prejudice against sufferers-locking all kinds of people away, controlling them as alienists did in Yorke and

---

[114] Berrios.G.E. Melancholia and Depression During the 19th Century: A Conceptual History. The British Journal of Psychiatry. Vol. 153. Issue 3. Sept.1988. 298.304.

[115] https://collections.nlm.nih.gov/catalog/nlm:nlmuid-28430960R-bk

[116] Scull, Andrew. C. Madhouses, Mad-Doctors and Madmen. The Social History of Psychiatry in the Victorian Era: University of Pennsylvania Press.

[117] http://www.studymore.org.uk/asyarc.htm

Bicetre. The buildings were both imposing and forbidding, creating their own environment, their own separate communities, representing also the industrialisation of care.

Summed up, the 19th century view of madness concerned self-absorption, or egotism, while sanity was object-related, looking out onto the material world and prizing it. This indeed is the world of the practical businessman, John Galsworthy, or his creation Soames, rather than John Keats, Byron and Shelley, and to same degree may have been a reaction to the Romantics early in the century who emphasised feelings , introspection and of losing control.

Towards the end of the century psychiatrists began to view physical causes as mainly responsible for mental illness, as can be seen in the disease construct. Their knowledge of physical diseases was limited by modern understanding, knowing nothing then of viruses, but believing that it simply appeared like a bad cold or small pox. Viruses were not known until Dimitri Ivanovski in 1892, but it was not until much later that the activity of viruses was understood. The causes were from birth or inherited and was linked in thought or intention with phrenology. The accepted idea of bad air or miasma seems an unlikely rationale, although some doctors or commentators held environment played a part, insisting that hospitals should be located in natural and beautiful parts of suburbia. They certainly did not believe it was caused by families as, contrary to reason, they tended to be regarded as good, even when bad and harmful.

Like ordinary physical illnesses mental illness often simply happened. At approximately the same time bloodletting was still debated as to its role in treating mental illness.[118]As has been noted, especially by Foucault [119], the method of cure was perceived as through the Superintendent's personality, his charisma and will. The sense of individual psychiatrists as providing the magical ingredients of cure is observable even now. The psychiatrist's personality delivered the ideology which provided the escape from confusion, the source of magic and cures (Foucault: 1965). Case studies invariably feature the doctor as a powerful efficacious intelligence, often breaking through ignorance to make stubborn patients aware of their madness-which often has been concluded by the doctor before an interview begins.

One factor in the past continues today: the dissonance between the high-toned and apparently complex (at times) thinking and communication of psychiatrists and their treatment practices, which were often barbaric but also indifferent to results. In the past, as now was a tendency to make huge claims for treatments that to outsiders seemed unjustified. It is likely that no one during this period, in fact throughout the history of the profession was cured with many lives made worse. The abiding sense is pursuit of psychiatric status with patients employed mainly as cannon fodder, one of the perceivable attitudes of elite groups at the time towards the poor and victimised. Although Foucault sees doctors as engaging in ideological battle with patients, in fact much of it concerned a profound sense of class and educational superiority.

---

[118] Pliny Earle.An Examination Practice of Bloodletting for Mental Disorders.
[119] Madness and Civilisation.
https://monoskop.org/images/1/14/Foucault_Michel_Madness_and_Civilization_A_History_of_Insanity_in_th
e_Age_of_Reason.pdf

By the end of the 19th century psychiatry had become international, with each country's doctors sharing ideas. Those of the USA were mirrored in Britain and in other parts of Europe. In 1820 [120]the Danes built their first asylum and the inmates were expected to engage in 'sporty' activities and checks were made on their moral character-that they avoided idleness, egotism, and any selfish vice that clearly only the insane suffered from not those treating them. In the mad these moral values would affect patients in extremis, inducing possible hysteria.[121]These problems were indeed put down to want of will-power and indolence, a union of selfishness and moral deceptivity (82), referencing indeed the mad as stubborn non-participants in the industrial society around them where work itself carried considerable moral values. Foucault notes Tuke's belief in work as an essential indication of sanity, a view still held by psychiatrists and gleaned from the works of Locke,[122] his views expressed in his Social Contract on the nature of the individual through citizenship, with specific responsibilities, and his views on human identity as separate and autonomous. Madness then was lacking autonomy, as expressed through citizen tropes of family, work and understanding. Strangely, given his more complex views on human experience, Freud believed the same.

Psychiatrists' lack of status:

Although there was recognition of some psychiatrists, Maudsley for example, the status for the majority remained low. The hospital environment institutionalised both patients and staff, as well as creating an experimental and liminal environment. The latter remains a psychological and intellectual issue for the profession as a whole as the processes through and in which they work has created its own reality, a false reality from which psychiatry issues its resolutions. This lack of reality stems from the absence of interaction between physicians and those they attempt to cure, the hierarchical element which encourages overreaching individual claims by psychiatrist regarding their intellects and knowledge and a shoring up of immense individual power.

In the old asylums the superintendent had:

1. Complete control of those under them
2. Were in positions in effect of monarchs or dictators, even often benign ones
3. Superintendents did little real observation but managed the facilities
4. Observation was done through a system of peer communication that was no more than anecdotal. Foucault perceives it correctly as a form of control.
5. The patients were not real people, simply descriptions, categories and behaviour traits.
6. In some measure, they defined themselves in opposition to how they defined patients. Patients were incapable of cognition, were animalistic and infantile. Often they were alien, the other. The doctors were of superior intelligence, if in fact themselves, in the end, strange.

---

[120] Stevenson, Christine. Madness and the Picturesque in the kingdom of Denmark. Bynum, Porter, Shepherd. The Anatomy of Madness. Essays in the History of Psychiatry. Vol. 111. The Asylum and its Psychiatry. Routledge. 2004. Page 82.

[121] Stevenson, Christine. Madness and the Picturesque in the kingdom of Denmark. Bynum, Porter, Shepherd. The Anatomy of Madness. Essays in the History of Psychiatry. Vol. 111. The Asylum and its Psychiatry. Routledge. 2004. Page 82.

[122] An Essay Concerning Human Understanding.

Hospital environments were cut off from the rest of the world, and so were the people in it and its thinking. Within such an environment, the belief in widespread mental illness within the negative, disease concept of psychiatry (read the DSM for continued confirmation of this) grew perceptively. As psychiatrist did not then, nor now engage with other disciplines it constructed ideas on human nature out of its own pathologies.

Other changes had ensued: state involvement in the management of the mentally ill with psychiatrists as state factotums, serving to seclude and control the mad. According to Scull,[123] it had become accepted that madness could be authoritatively diagnosed, treated and certified by an elite group of legally recognised experts. The defining of psychiatry through law connected them to other middle-class elites. Treatment became official and authorised. *Nobody not deemed an expert could officially treat a mentally ill person, even though being an expert seems similar to being part of a group or club, where rituals are undergone in order to be part of that group or club. Believing the dominant ideology, the biological argument, helps but is not essential.*

Scull describes an ideological battle towards the end of the century between Neurologists, who located madness in the brain, those who responded to Moral Therapy, devising a mixture of the two, including within the general armoury phrenology (page 8). It must also be remembered that paradigms of race, colonialism, reflected in the expansion of psychiatry, and eugenics whereby faulty humans could be dispensed with or treated harshly were constituents. Into the general vigorous pool (Scull: page 8) was thrown in an American-based obsession with cure-that is every patient, where possible, should be cured. This represented and still represents an ideal, an un-validated paradigm that suggests another desirable state exists beyond the individual's state. While this may be desirable where criminal consequences are involved, it carries with it ideological and intellectual problems that psychiatry as a whole largely deals with by ignoring it and substituting group efficacy-*I know best*-for evidence or analysis.

In this argument, Scull does not present the philosophical stance of Henry Maudsley who stood out against what he and many of his generation saw as the vague misplaced humanitarism of Moral Treatment and were intent on replacing it with evolutionary biology and degeneration theory, creating thereby a different kind of fuzziness. His generation, perhaps taking a lead from Pinel, instituted observation as a means of acquiring proper data on mental illness, the kind of information that could be used for reports and articles. Maudsley made his reputation through his articles that, as I have noted, helped popularise the case study as a means of conveying mental health ideas to his peers in psychiatry and the greater world beyond.[124]

Maudsley's efforts in clinical journalism helped to create the psychiatric profession, establishing its monopoly in the administration and care of the mentally ill. This was a process that today seems triumphant but not perhaps healthy. Free of competition, domination of any discipline quickly becomes dogma and of course liable to institutionalise abuse. Psychiatry, through the efforts of Maudsley and his generation, became the accepted clinical approach to

---

[123] Madhouses, Mad-Doctors and Madmen: The Social History of Psychiatry in the Victorian era. University of Pennsylvania Press. 1981.

[124]Davie, Niel. *"False in Doctrine and Cruel in Practice." Henry Maudsley the M'naghten Rules and and Mental Responsibility.* Unpublished paper. 2011. Universitie Lumiere Lyon. Academia edu.

mental illness and its notions of control and paternalism natural to the care of those judged insane.

It was not until the 1860s that psychiatrists became a fixture in mental hospitals, a situation Maudsley helped create with his journalism and assertive views. Yet, psychiatry remained intellectually unconvincing, the profession tending to throw out judgements on causation like darts at a moving object. Mental illness had something to do with the brain, its causes were clearly physical, falling back on the descriptive narratives found in the DSM, basing mental illness on character and as noted phrenology.

The important factors were, it would appear, the accreditation, influence and power of the psychiatric profession and the dominance of their viewpoints fashioned in isolation in asylums.[125]

5.

By 1900 the rise of dynamic psychiatry, exampled by people like Freud, began to overtake the somatic psychiatry of the previous century, which now of course is dominant again. Freud's philosophical understanding and adventurous intellectualism gave energy and interest to mental illness that lasted until the 1960s before being swamped by laboratory psychiatry that remains dominant. In the meantime, asylums flourished and completely ignored dynamic psychiatry inventing instead new or reinvigorating old ways to attack both body and brain.

A major difference between somatic understandings of mental illness and dynamic understandings is the comparative crudity of thought of the former combined with historical paradigms of categorisation and control. Although not much evident in asylums, under dynamic psychiatry the patient became an important collaborative and identified part of the cure not simply an object, as in somatic therapy, to be worked on by largely self-appointed experts. Where Freud developed a map of the mind, most psychiatrists saw mental illness as functioning on a flat horizon and the human patient as resembling a fractured machine or lower animal. The fact that there was some evidence that dynamic psychiatry worked for some patients, nevertheless it took time and was expensive. It was unlikely therefore to last when faced with relatively cheaper and industrial forms of therapy, and a profession claiming again its dominance. Even moral therapy required a little too much brain power for many psychiatrists who simply had managerial rather than psychological skills combined with an elites' sense of entitlement.

Pagel declared in an edited text of *Introduction to the History of Medicine*1915 that Pinel alleged that mental illness was a disease like any other (sic), bringing his views back to the ideology of physicians [126], described above, a view that continued alongside Freud's psychodynamic views and was peculiar to *Asylum Psychiatry* and aspects of *Office Psychiatry* where all mental health problems followed the pattern of diagnosis (often without co-operation)-prescription (drugs)-claims of cure that again are not necessarily corroborated by patients or evidenced in their own lives. Psychiatry's perception of a cure is a negative one and

---

[125] Davie, Niel. *"False in Doctrine and Cruel in Practice."* Henry Maudsley the M'naghten Rules and and Mental Responsibility. Unpublished paper. 2011. Universitie Lumiere Lyon. Academia edu.
[126] Ed. Micale, Mark S/Porter, Roy. Discovering the History of Psychiatry. Oxford University Press. 1994.

usually they do not expect patients to overcome their problems, diseases can often have no clear causation after all, but to not feel or think abnormally. For psychiatry, a cure means not thinking at all. The only times psychiatrist's accept or enable achievement is when or if an achievement happens the patient continues to depend on them and continues to routinely accept their own mental illness.

Part 2 of this survey begins at approximately 1950 with the rise again of somatic psychiatry based on drug therapy, the monoamine hypothesis, DSM and personality disorder. As this paper comes to a close its assertions can be itemised as:

1) The influence and power of psychiatry and its development throughout the 19th century.

2) Its creation of clinical ideas in isolation

3) The character based nature of its ideas with a connection to Phrenology.

4) Its vague claims to the physical causes of mental illness

5) Psychiatrists' monopolisation of both the running of and ideas behind mental health.

Part 2: Intellectual history of Psychiatry.

20th Century Psychiatry-Present

By late 1950s,[127] reliance on crude, non-scientific interventions (e.g. lobotomy andinsulin coma therapy), had been replaced by chemical interventions (e.g. largactil[chlorpromazine] and imipramine) which raised unrealistic hope of cure.

Many see 20th century psychiatry as being a contest between *dynamic psychiatry* (the mind) and *somatic psychiatry* (physical origins of mental illness), but it can equally be understood as between different interactive processes; the former attempts an understanding of how different conditions can be negotiated via the therapist as conduit of knowledge and insight, while Asylum based psychiatry places emphasis on hierarchies-the doctor is always right and their position is based on power. The doctor's therapeutic perspective is contained by diagnosis and is usually restricted to drug prescriptions. There is insufficient evidence that either is effective. Both developed out of Moral Treatment but the latter preserved the dictatorial powers and largely ideological viewpoint that while it has its rationale in Pinel, gains much of its energy from Victorian Medical Superintendents and their day to day focus on extreme instances of mental illness.

While Asylum Psychiatry formats have changed, residing now in *Laboratory* or *Biological Psychiatry*, the methods of delivery have not. For the present, *Laboratory Psychiatry* with its dogma of biological aetiology of illness is perceived as correct, mainly because of the increased dominance of medical doctors in modern society and, in line with Joanna Moncrieff's understanding, its intensive popularisation via the media. The idea of '*wonder drugs*', which I have attempted to show is the obverse of the real situation, has gained thereby manifest currency.[128] The laissez faire approach of *Dynamic Psychiatry* is perhaps less desired in driven, conformist and corporate societies where stress and confusion can be dealt with by the immediacy and accessibility of drugs. Psychiatric, here mainly referencing *Asylum Psychiatry*, monopolisation of the mental illness discourse has occurred over approximately the last 150 years and therefore is not as embedded in treatments as often imagined.

Unfortunately, *Asylum Psychiatry* dominance brings with it crudity of thinking and often of methods. It has through Monoamine Hypothesis reduced the human brain to the level of a rat and largely, but not entirely, extinguished the mind. Strangely, people have colluded with this process allowing for the existence of a strange dichotomy-high cognitive and imaginative concepts routinely discussed on mind and consciousness and the primitive reductionism of psychiatry dealing with the main contributory organ-the brain. Rather than discuss the views in relation to mental illness (a much more doubtful concept than routinely accepted) with reference to Jung, Penrose, Freud, and John Searle generally people have embraced the claims of chemists concerned mainly with gathering profits.[129]

---

[127] Yoganathan, N. /Dr J Willis. The Madness of Psychiatry (in 21st Century UK): Large Group Analytic Perspective

[128] The Psychoactive Effects of Psychiatric Medication: The Elephant in the Room Joanna Moncrieff M.B.B.S. , David Cohen & Sally Porter. 2013.A

[129] Yes, a crude estimate in itself but unfortunately closer to the truth than people realise.

Asylum Psychiatry positioned the mentally ill as the *Other*[130], those locked away (behind walls or the effects of drugs), categorised and controlled by a single elite group, with a persistent dynamic of expansion in order to achieve legitimacy. Opposition has mainly dried up. Warnings about its ideas and practices tossed into the wind, fluttering away beyond the grasp of both ordinary citizens and the powers-that-be, the latter tending anyway to respond to its simplistic arguments and power tropes. Interestingly, *Asylum Psychiatry* developed many modern forms of torture such as water-boarding. As with other forms of psychiatry, *Asylum Psychiatry* functions within its own rules, often indifferent to the laws and codes of society, happily subjecting young children to invasive treatments while diagnosing the vulnerable without concern for repercussions, harassing those it has categorised as mentally ill.

Upon briefly detailing the history of psychiatry from the turn of the century this paper will provide a number of often clashing views on present psychiatry. It will hope to identify why the failings of *Asylum Psychiatry*, its ideology and practices, are being so assiduously ignored. It will also suggest that evidence of success of psychiatric treatment is down to the placebo effect and is despite treatments given.

History

Although the common view is that *Dynamic Psychiatry*, with its inclination towards philosophy and focus on the mind, was dominant in the first half of the last century, *Asylum Psychiatry* was the main service provider, with the number of people it dealt with noticeably subject to increase. It offered protection for the severely mentally ill while at the same time confirming their separate, alien nature. Under the auspices of *Asylum Psychiatry* the mentally ill were viewed as odd and dangerous, while in *Dynamic Psychiatry* they were merely viewed as different with the positives examined and sometimes celebrated. The ideology of cure affects both disciplines, but with *Asylum Psychiatry* it came in spasms and involved invasive treatments such as ECT and lobotomy-treatments capable of permanently harming patients- all based on very little science. Nevertheless *Asylum Psychiatry* dealt also with the brain damaged, and Alzheimer patients where perhaps often its ideologies proved efficacious. The dictatorial powers of psychiatrists as noted formed from these areas.

Asylum Psychiatry has long been a profession searching desperately- for ideological, status and economic reasons-for scientific justification. This was a common process for the medical profession as a whole, up until the present. In mental health this was clearly in preference to just being managers of the mad, the main activity prior to the Yorke Retreat and Pinel's Bicetre and indeed afterwards until the 1950s.

Up to that point, *Asylum Psychiatry* produced its worst abuses and was deserving of its bad reputation, while still taking in vulnerable adults and children at the behest of parents and spouses without even a backward glance at state laws. This paper will look at two, one of which continued until recently.

Lobotomy:

---

[130] A reasonable sociological term.

Lobotomy emerged out of the decade of fascist states and extreme nationalism, and through its absolutism, violence and ferocity reflected both. Devised first in Portugal by Antonio Caetano de Abreu Freire "Egas" Moniz in 1935, it arrived in the United States in 1936-about the time the western world began once again to experience extreme violence. The principal operation involved separating fibres connecting the frontal lobes to the thalamus. Less common at first was the transorbital lobotomy that involved an instrument shaped like an icepick being hammered through the orbital plate (eyesocket) and moved back and forward to the same effect. This was one, but only one, of the extreme devices of Asylum Psychiatry possible because in this form of psychiatric medicine people could be forced to undergo whatever treatments the doctor deemed suitable. Devoid of the freedoms of autonomy (in doctors' eyes) patients were merely available fodder. The connection here between Asylum Psychiatry and infamous Nazi doctors who experimented on concentration camp victims is perhaps both too close for comfort and too obvious to ignore. Tens of thousands of men, women and children, according to Jenell Johnson[131], not unconnected in effect to the present day psychiatric practice of giving drugs to 6 year olds, for example, through the radical uncontrolled labelling children with AHDH diagnosis and other dubious appellations. As with drug-treatments, the operation was held as heralding 'a golden age of discovery and healing.'(Jenell: 2013: 2), and its inventor, Moniz, given the Nobel Prize for Medicine in 1949. The passage below, written in 1942, replicates the praise of biological psychiatric remedies:

The treatment of mental disorders has undergone a number of changes in the past two decades. Some of these changes have come to stay, others have been thoroughly tested out and are being restricted or discarded, and still others are just beginning to be investigated. The gratifying results of the malaria therapy for paresis have been followed by the formidable shock methods of treatment with insulin and metrazol, and by the vitamin treatment of the deficiency disorders. The surgical treatment of mental disorders is still in its infancy, and in offering this volume the authors have endeavored to establish a foundation for future work along the same lines. They recognize only too well their own limitations in dealing with such a complex subject as the relationship between the brain and mental disease, yet they have attempted to present the facts, to do justice to past work in the field, and to speculate with one foot occasionally upon the ground. They are inclined to agree with the original concept that the frontal lobes are essential for satisfactory social adaptation; but they suggest that certain individuals may suffer from perverted activity of these areas and may become capable of better adaptation when these lobes are partially inactivated. Theories are developed concerning the mechanism by which the perverted activity of the frontal lobes produces deviation in behavior; and the conclusion is reached that without the frontal lobes there could be no functional psychoses. Perhaps this is an extreme view, perhaps it is only self-evident. Partial separation of the frontal lobes from the rest of the brain results in reduction of disagreeable self-consciousness, abolition of obsessive thinking, and satisfaction with performance, even though the performance is inferior in quality. The emotional nucleus of the psychosis is removed, the "sting" of the disorder, is drawn. Even though the fixed ideas persist and the compulsions continue for a while, the fear that disabled the patient is banished. How much this relief means to the patient suffering from doubts and

---

[131] American Lobotomy. A Rhetorical History. University of Michigan Press. Ann Arbour. 2013.

fears, morbid thoughts, hallucinations and delusions, and compulsive activities, may easily be imagined.[132]

Analysing the language, because rarely done, is important here. Many active words are employed: shock, problems are removed and drawn. The physical nature of treatments are underlined demonstrating that the doctor has to exert themselves to acquire results. In fact, the active verbs as a whole are violent or indicate possible violence. Perverted is used several times, distinguishing perhaps the physicians' reaction to pathology, but also underlining the sexual nature, principally disgust, of the thinking. The *self-conscious* is disagreeable. As I have before pointed out, in modern psychiatry everything is perceived of as negative.

Many of the patients who underwent the above procedures would probably have been coerced.

In America, the operation continued until the 1950s in, it must be supposed, contradiction of all acceptable western values.[133] Psychiatrists had by then discovered another 'sure' science-drugs. So, effectively, one act which if performed by ordinary citizens would be considered barbaric and criminal was followed by another which if otherwise pursued in the backstreets of modern cities would have been and is considered criminal. Freeman, one of the authors of the above paper, actually and infamously employed an icepick on hundreds of patients, and also on a 12 year old boy.

These two acts (or multiplicity of acts) defined the separation between Asylum Psychiatry and *Laboratory* or *Biological Psychiatry*. Although Jenell insists it was not quite the horror story of slasher movies, nevertheless a 12 year old boy was operated on, see above. The reach of *Asylum Psychiatry* was actually ameliorated by drug treatments even though the same vocabulary is erroneously employed for both in psychiatry's desire for respectability and the status of a science.

The second dangerous remedy considered here was and is Electric Convulsive Therapy, or ECT, a treatment given widely that caused temporary cures of depression but damaged memory and cognition. [134]Invented in 1938, it has a high rate of relapse and appears, where it is successful, to provide temporary relief. There is continued uncertainty about how it works, when it does,[135] and the uncertainty over[136]its side effects. Although some authorities claim that ECT does not affect brain-damage, this again is not the information I gained from my clients [137] and again independent research seems necessary. Nowadays, at least some information services provide accurate information, a result probably of the patients'

---

[132] Freeman, W., Watts, J. W., & Hunt, T. (Collaborator). (1942). Psychosurgery: Intelligence, emotion, and social behavior following prefrontal lobotomy for mental disorders. London, England: Baillière, Tindall & Cox.

[133] https://jamanetwork.com/journals/archneurpsyc/article-abstract/650027

[134] Fink/Nemeroff. *The Neuroendocrine View of ECT*. Convulsive Therapy. 5 (3):296-304. 1989. Raven Press Ltd.

[135] Weiner, et al. American Psychiatric Association. Committee on Electroconvulsive Therapy. The practice of electroconvulsive therapy: recommendations for treatment, training and privileging. Washington DC. American Psychiatric Publishing. 2001.

[136]://www.academia.edu/26790462/Manic_reactions_to_ECT://www.academia.edu/26790462/Manic_reactio n/

[137] https://www.swedish.org/services/behavioral-health/our-services/electroconvulsive-therapy

movements of the 1990s.[138] As a treatment, it has been used since the 1940s but in the 1950s-60s it was used extensively and employed over-vigorously often without consent. This was indeed a period of psychiatrist dominance and subjectivity, without necessary safeguards against physician egotism (are there ever many?).[139]

Although statements from patients given ECT must not override the dangers of the treatment, which too often are ignored by physicians or are part of a gamble involving patients' long term health.[140] Charlotte Blease is one academic who considers the benevolent effects are unproven and fit more the placebo effect when such results occasionally do appear[141]. *Asylum Psychiatry* remains (perhaps) the only medical discipline that can damage patients' health irredeemably, and which has already left several cohorts of destroyed lives. There are several works on the matter, from my *An Unusual Power*, which is incomplete and does not include the late Victorian period when *Asylum Psychiatry* became more determined to prove itself and thereby damaged patients' more severely, and *A Mad People's History of Madness* by Dale Peterson, which provides missing data and focuses on false imprisonment in asylums that continued until the 1990s in slightly different forms.[142] A more recent book detailing modern abuse is Linda Andre's *Doctors of Deception: What they don't want you to know about shock treatment*[143] which concentrates more on ECT and backs up my deep concerns about its use.

A more in-depth piece of research by Lucy Johnstone highlights the ignorance of patients regarding ECT, although there is much more information now, and she suggests some of the misunderstanding might be due to patient memory loss. A number of patients expressed approval of ECT but unlike many recent surveys Johnstone looked behind the original results. She found patient fear of rejection or worse by the psychiatric staff if they expressed negative views towards the treatment. She expressed the view that this phenomenon might affect other mental health patient surveys. Patients only gave their real opinions when they trusted the researcher (71). Researchers were apparently surprised, in several surveys gathered by the author, in many clearly frightened patients compliance with ECT, which they put down to resignation rather than coercion. Nevertheless such behaviour it does reflect a heightened degree of helplessness when faced with doctor's demands. A small number of patients, perhaps the most honest, were hostile towards it and/or deeply frightened.

Any research done by researchers outside the system reflects a wholly negative response. Such research is usually provides honest rather than self-fulfilling results. One survey done by UKAN[144], Mindlink and Survivors Speak Out (the last two service users organisations) revealed that 35% believed ECT was damaging and another 16% suggested it was unhelpful; some 30% had positive views while the remainder employed words like 'brutal' and 'barbaric'. Psychological after-effects, hardly ever recorded in official surveys probably to the surprise of

---

[138] http://www.healthtalk.org/peoples-experiences/mental-health/electroconvulsive-treatment/side-effects-having-ect

[139] https://www.mind.org.uk/information-support/drugs-and-treatments/electroconvulsive-therapy-ect/#.W-LynfZ2tMs

[140] https://www.bbc.com/news/health-23414888

[141] ECT. The Importance of Informed consent and the 'Placebo Literacy'. Journal of Medical Ethics 2012 10.1136/medethics-2012-101201

[142] University of Pittsburgh Press. 1982.

[143] Rutgers University Press. 2009.

[144] UK Advocacy Nationwide.

many unused to the service, pointed to a drop in confidence and self-esteem. *Coercion was found to occur in a number of cases (page 74).*

The evidence above has to be considered in the light of the Royal College of Psychiatrists declaration (1997) that there was no evidence that ECT harmed patients, and the assertions of patients and observers that doctors were not interested in patients' views on the matter. There has been a recent move back towards ECT, its benefits insisted on by a number of papers that breach standards of research in that only initial behaviour and comments are sought and looked for. The thoughts and feelings of patients are still rarely canvased.

Asylum Psychiatry's Triumph

The dominance of somatic or *Asylum Psychiatry* appeared over the horizon of 1950 perhaps as a side product of military experiments with drugs on their enemy and their own soldiers, the growth of chemical companies and their place in the economy and the lastly the paradigm of mental illness as a disease which necessitated drug treatment in line with drugs as the preferable method of treatment for a variety of diseases.

This also applies to probably the best-known attempt to dispose of classic narratives – and at the same time their subject. Edward Shorter's history of psychiatry (1997) – which to a certain extent assesses development over the past decades from the other side of the institutional landscape – notes an end to psychiatry that manifests itself in the disintegration of psychiatric pathology, in the success of psychopharmacology, in the separation of the psychodynamic through neurophysiological explanatory models and, last but not least, in the end of classic institutional treatment.[145]

Although the shutting down of asylums or mental hospitals was conceived at the highest levels, drug treatments would have ensured that end. The necessity of controlling patients was gone once they could receive drugs, possibly known early on to be addictive, allowing a close eye to be kept on patients from the first point of contact, General Practitioners, an essential quality of *Asylum Psychiatry*- that is its policing activities.

Clorpromazine, the first anti-psychotic, was initially produced as an antihistaminergic by the French pharmaceutical company Rohne-Poulenc, it was for use against nausea and allergies. Experiments on rats demonstrated that it had a calming effect, and given to patients before surgeries again demonstrated tranquillising effects.[146]Further tests on patients indicated again

---

[145] Hess, Majerus. Writing the History of Psychiatry in the 20th Century. Article *in* History of Psychiatry · June 2011
DOI: 10.1177/0957154X11404791 · Source: PubMed

[146] https://www.bap.org.uk/articles/chlorpromazine-the-first-antipsychotic

a calming tendency that was seen in their decreased anxiety and calm behaviour. Such drugs are given nowadays by dentists for example and often but not always produced sedative effects-as most such drugs do including heroin of course and marihuana. That is why or one reason many recreational drugs are taken. The subsequent spread of its use was the result of SmithKline & French, the licence holders, who ran a brilliant marketing campaign.

The claims since for the success of psychopharmacology is remarkable for its florid self-endorsements-for example from the British Association for Psychopharmacology-[147]which is not reflected in many authoritative articles. Edward Kouassi[148] asserts that valuation of efficacy is based on indirect evidence and Shorter (1997) flawed assessment design. The results of tests are always without fail down to the estimate of the observer, often a clinician, and are thereby corrupted by predicted outcomes. Tests done in a culture of conviction, as most RCTs are, can assumed to be corrupted, and what occurs is a valuation of drug performance according to the dynamics of drug actions on the body, not their efficacy on psychosis.[149] The paper referenced at this point discusses the efficacy of Clorpromazine and other antipsychotics without mentioning human beings throughout, restricting everything to drug actions. A valid confirmation of the term *Laboratory Psychiatry*. Unfortunately, research that denies the validity of psychotropic drugs are drummed out in the routine avalanche of papers that simply repeat the group's entrenched position.

Capitalism:

The essential part played by capitalism should not be played down. Notwithstanding its good or bad effects, the process of developing a product and then a market for it seems conspicuous here, and is common in pharmaceutical companies and psychiatry making it hard to see the joins. The tranquillising effect of such drugs did not necessarily go beyond that and had an effect on how the patient's psychosis affected them, not the illness. A problem with this economic model is that more customers/patients must be found and more illnesses discovered for more products.

---

[147] https://www.bap.org.uk/articles/a-brief-history-of-psychiatric-drug-development/

[148] www.thelancet.com Vol 382 December 7, 2013

[149] Samara. M.T. et al. Clorpromazine versus every other antipsychotic for Schizophrenia: A systematic review and meta-analysis challenging.....European Neuropsychopharmacology 2014.

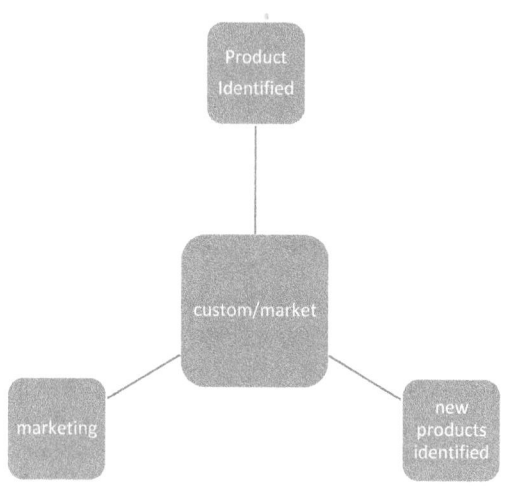

The market/customers need to then be increased and new custom identified and new, if similar, products produced by identifying new markets or similar but sufficiently different ones. Thereby depression, for example, can be fragmented into degrees of difficulty and drug compounds identified to meet each fragment-let's say Depression level b and Depression level c. [150]

In this model, more and more people are diagnosed with depression. There are more workers employed in mental health and more clinics and other services provided. The drugs are merely created from similar compounds to the first compound, often just branded with different names. More and more people seem to suffer from mental illness, more drugs are sold, and *Asylum Psychiatry* expands its status and power. The creation of asylums, as noted, had before vastly increased the number being diagnosed.

Specialists emerge who are familiar with Depression level b, and those familiar with Depression level c. Some specialists would be familiar with both. The latter may be particularly brilliant and design further levels all contained within their own form within the construct of Depression, but without context. If context is added, which it never is, Depression c and b, for example appear very different. Depression b might concern someone losing their employment

---

[150] This actually occurs.

and Depression c might appear after the unemployment continues and hope is lost. The drug companies do not itemise reasons, they are concerned only with affects.

The emergence of Clorpromazine is curious in so much as the tranquillising effects of plants and the drugs often obtained from them have been recognised for several thousand years, so to label this a breakthrough lacks credence. What was a breakthrough was the production of such a drug in bulk saleable form, easily transported and marketed. Additional reasons for its success were the creation of National Health services after the 2nd World War, functioning as corporates with ease of communication/information, movement of personnel, close association of education of its workforce and top-down ideologies-the education of doctors requires a mechanistic approach to treatments and therefore students unwilling to challenge perceived wisdom; initiatives on health by the United Nations and its concern with the health of individuals and the right to health-driving cures; the provision of stable and lucrative work for all systemically qualified doctors in National Health Services (UK: 1948) creating a homogeneous mass of physicians, the good and bad physicians no longer identified. These changes facilitated the rapid acceptance of psychotropic drugs. The continued production required an increased supply of patients (the extension of mental illness noticeable in the DSM and through constructs of Anxiety and Depression), and new mental illnesses to accompany and encourage this expansion.

To emphasise, the creation and testing of these drugs are laboratory based without even a nod to human consumption. The subjective experiences of *consumers* are not recorded only the clinicians' evaluations. Moncrieff, Cohen and Mason (2009) produced data taken from internet sites on which patients wrote freely (most patients are too intimidated by their doctors to voice concerns)[151] and produced these conclusions:

Cognitive impairment

Emotional flattening

Depressive and suicidal feelings (by some)

Societal Consequence:

A number of physical effects were noted. Cognitive impairment covered a range including decision making and judgement. The lack of feeling was noted by all, or practically so. This is a common complaint of psychotropic drugs. These kind of reactions are likely to be produce a range of experiential conditions-inability to feel and take responsibility for example-that over time would create personality disorders-constantly denied by psychiatrists. On such drugs many kinds of behaviour are possible, neglect of family, errant behaviour and worse. SSRIs are, this paper insists, responsible for criminal behaviour. A combination of euphoria, reported by many, and inability to have emotions or emotional responses, reported by most, would probably encourage grandeur and recklessness.

---

[151] The subjective experience of taking anti-psychotic medication: a content analysis of internet data. Acta Psychiatr Scand 2009: 120: 102–111 All rights reserved DOI: 10.1111/j.1600-0447.2009.01356.x Wiley Pub.

Some people recorded benefits from the above symptoms, but again this is in line with recreational drugs regular intake.

The use of psychoactive drugs often causes criminal behaviour for some of the reasons noted above, initiating lower levels of connectedness to others through effects on the user's emotions. Personality changes can be noted. It seems highly unlikely therefore that personality alteration does not occur with long-term users of psychotropic drugs.[152]Commonly reported effects are euphoria, as with psychotropic drugs, and paranoia.

By mass-producing drugs, mass custom was and is also required to make economic sense of the health industry; individuals are then a commodity, their health subject to economic prosperity brought and sold. The more money goes through the system usually the healthier an economy is, with, in Britain, the National Health Service acting as part of the central money focus (value, not cash) its abstracted and concrete forms going around like blood through veins. Mental health is essential in this process, because unlike physical health which is finite (a broken leg can be broken in many places with associated difficulties and diagnosis but there is a defined number of both), mental health remains an abstraction which can be added to, fragmented and restructured. Today Depression, tomorrow something else of a similar nature. The monoamine hypothesis provides a one shoe fits all approach, without individual causality, making it easier to treat (or appear to treat) people. It is a mass diagnosis for the masses, with mass produced treatments.

Since the invention, production and marketing of chlorpromazine *Asylum/Laboratory Psychiatry* has expanded its base and *Dynamic* or mind psychiatry has become the lesser cousin. It has become accepted that mental illness has a biological base, constructed on experiments with mice and rats, and templates that have excluded the mind, intentionality, thought, hope and desire as development paradigms and given even greater power to psychiatry. The number employed is now far greater than those employed under *dynamic psychiatry*. Human beings are now ciphers directed by the will of powerful psychiatrists who are close to having the powers denied to them in the 19th century. A little after the discovery of chlorpromazine the DSM was constructed containing descriptive if doubtful examples of mental illness with its inclination towards moral urgency. This was an essential step taken by Asylum medicine that enabled it to expand into public consciousness and gain prominence and power within society itself-although it would not have been expressed in that fashion but within professional vision and ethic tropes. The second step in this expansion was the monoamine hypothesis that provided a scientific description of the effects of drugs allowing a growing acceptance of *Biological* or *Laboratory Psychiatry*. The latter appellation well describes present psychiatry as all the evidence produced comes from laboratory research on animals. Further developments of the DSM and growing acceptance of personality disorder, a handy tool which is so flexible and fluid that its calculations can fit anyone-and everyone. If you work too hard, you are mentally ill, if you work too little, you are mentally ill, if you love too many

[152] Newcombe, Russell. Psychonautics:A Model and Method for Exploring the Subjective Effects of Psychoactive drugs. #d Research Bureau. 1999.
https://pdfs.semanticscholar.org/6a56/7f9995f20655ce950aa0cff393934cc0e0a2.pdf

women or men, or too few, the same applies, if you exercise too much you are mentally ill, too little and the same can apply.

Several expansions of the DSM have occurred and more apparent confirmation of monoamine (first accepted in the 1960s) causation for mental illness, and with it, unsurprisingly perhaps, more people with mental illness identified. [153] Philosophical and epistemic concerns are routinely raised about the DSM, as here, but as routinely ignored. Rarely do psychiatrists worry over the essential nature of mental illness, convinced by the authenticity of their training. Psychiatrists have continued to exalt the[154] wonder drugs and ignore patient complaints or query their actual affects. [155]

Originally, as considered by Moncrieff et al (2013), antipsychotic drugs were referred to as *chemical coshes*, useful in controlling patients while smothering their feelings, and tranquillisers were called '*mother's little helpers*', referencing their similar squashing of mood swings that were a distinctive part of grappling with living on post-war council estates in which community connections had broken down or been removed, living dreary lives without hope. They were thereby employed to control the general population, given out by GPs like charitable sweet suppliers engaged by governments to keep disappointed children quiet. The over-prescribing of tranquillisers during mass unemployment in the 1980s is further evidence of this tendency. They had no other purpose. Now psychiatrists describe the same drugs as possessing discrete and sophisticated qualities; not just that but each one has identifiable results on different stages of depression and anxiety. Different effects or different brands? Coupled with these novel assertions, the same drugs are in contradiction versatile.

The serotonin basis of depression, while not easily dismissed, suffers from lack of definite proof and clarification as to the process after the triggering effect. Are all neurones affected, or at least a sufficient number, at the same time and if so how: is it a tsunami affect or sympathetic reactions over a greater period of time? Monoamine oxidase has been identified as a possible way to extend each phenomenon (single or in a group?) but any consideration has so far included maybes and perhaps in abundance-typical of the monoamine arguments. [156]The model given again presents the picture of monoamines working automatically and independently of the host, which (this is a human being) functions like a puppet at their instructions producing affects in a neutral world without cognition or intentionality. This is not the human world, but one invented by *Asylum Psychiatry*. The model posits a world within the brain that is not connected to the environment, but at the same time anthropomorphises the function of monoamines. Another paper insists it is about energy expended by neurones[157] and like an overworked electrical system can fail.

Recent research into the ways in which the brain functions has identified a communication effect between different parts of the brain, not related necessarily to any clear serotonin

---

[153] Cooper, Rachel.What is Wrong with the DSM?
https://journals.sagepub.com/doi/abs/10.1177/0957154X04039343
[154] http://news.bbc.co.uk/1/hi/health/1325629.stm
[155] www.dependency.net/learn/tranquiliser
[156] Richardson, JS. On the functions of monoamine oxidase, the emotions, and adaptation to stress.
International Journal of Neuroscience. May 1993. www.ncbi.nlm.nih.gov/pubmed/8083027
[157] www.sciencedirect.com/science/article/pii/so896627312007568

phenomenon, which according to the scientists involved produces sadness. [158] After recording brain activity transmitted by previously fitted electrodes the researchers found that 'conversation' occurred between the amygdala (thought to be responsible for emotions) and hippocampus (where memory is thought to reside). This appears to situate sadness within the memory of negative emotions, as Cognitive Behavioural Therapy claims, and also provides a mechanism for longer, deeper depressions. In fact parts of the oxidase model would fit this, except that this model offers acceptable levels of causation and stations any monoamine effect as a secondary function-where it belongs. This would provide a reason for the occasional short-term success of ECT, which the serotonin hypothesis does not. There has of course been attempts to connect the two practices-notably in 1989 (Fink and Nemeroff)[159]-which claims to detect the necessary neuroendocrine changes but stresses it is clinically based (a euphemism here for guess work) and not proven, and until tests are done on animals (rats?) they cannot be sure of their conclusions. As ECT produces regular negative effects on schizophrenia sufferers, worsening the condition, doubt must be thrown on much medical speculation.

While the serotonin phenomenon might be the way rats register stress and apathy (surely not with the complexity of human beings?), perhaps the former is the main method of human beings-fitting more what we know of the human brain. The use of mice and rats for research is apparently because like humans they manufacture endocrines, which researchers believe makes them most similar to humans. But all vertebrates manufacture endocrines.

Case Studies:

This paper began with one view of psychiatry. Another can be seen in Shrinks: the Untold Story of Psychiatry by Jeffrey A. Lieberman (and Ogi Ogas)[160], a leading psychiatrist of his day who affirms that this is a time of great new discoveries in psychiatry. Lieberman routinely attacks psychoanalysis, but provides only anecdotal evidence, often without clear additional evidence of the veracity of his claims to cures. While on the one hand he trounces the charlatanism of the more outlandish therapists such as Reich he appears, to an outsider, to function in much the same way. His first brilliant attempt at diagnosis is presented as a wonder of efficacy, but seems not to have been agreed with by others. Although he puts this down to other's ignorance (of which he clearly is not a victim), there is no further evidence that the young woman in question continued to suffer. Generally, the reader might believe his version (it is after all only his) because the process he recounts and expressions he employs might be believed in by his peers, who constitute a large number of state-supported individuals.

The parents of a university student complain to Leiberman that their daughter is continually distracted and has lost interest in her studies. They relate to him a recent incident where she

---

[158] https://www.livescience.com/64043-sadness-brain-activity.html?utm_source=ls-newsletter&utm_medium=email&utm_campaign=20181109-l
[159] Convulsive Therapy. 296-304. Raven Press Ltd. New York.
[160] Hachett UK, 2015.

met a dishevelled stranger in the street and goes back to his room with him. They are clearly concerned that something terrible might happen to her if such behaviour continues.

The doctor requests from the patient's parents the chance to interview her. Reluctantly, which the doctor puts down to a fear or distrust of psychiatry, they eventually agree but only after trying other kinds of treatment, each dismissed haughtily by Leiberman in the manner described earlier in *An Unusual Power* of university educated doctors deriding cunning people.

He has a short interview with her. He describes the girl as listless, her voice flat (one side effect, in fact, of anti-psychotic drugs). He further describes her as displaying narcissism, based on his assessment that she believes everything is about her, a common enough complaint of the young, These assessments appear to have their roots in *Asylum Psychiatry*, as when doctors began having regular, intimate knowledge of their patients they noted this quality. Freud did the same indicating patients' absorption in their problems. As Schizophrenia was not recorded until the outset of psychiatry the narcissism might have had something to do with medical practices or identified only later as an unusual, abnormal characteristic. Before it might have been accepted as just another human variation.

Her inability to focus on the interview the physician considers evidence of '*fragmented attention*'. Not perhaps boredom? It seems to Lieberman that the patient was attending to matters in her own mind and was indifferent to the environment. She speaks of great forces working through her and he then decides she is suffering, on one interview it appears, from schizophrenia. He informs her parents (not really concerned about any consequences to such a dramatic diagnosis) and persuades them into allowing him to provide their daughter with treatment. He places her on a Respiridone, a drug used for a number of proscribed illnesses and not just schizophrenia, has tests done to make sure no other causes are possible-but does not say exactly what they might be-and employs cognitive therapists for socialisation training. Respiridone is used for a wide number of conditions confirming Joanna Moncrieff's belief that such drugs function much the same within different brand names. Certainly they confirm psychiatric knowledge, corresponding to the educated wisdom of the few.

Lo, a miracle occurs. Unfortunately, her parents do not believe it has anything to do with his treatments or that a miracle has even occurred. Her parent's views are of course dismissed.

They decide not to let their daughter continue with him. It is not to do with perhaps his sense of superiority, his dogmatic approach and that he holds that at all times he knows better of course? We only have his side here.

What possible problems are there here; he provides no evidence that once rejecting his therapy the girl has any further problems; that his approach may have alienated the parents and girl; he stresses that the girl is better because she becomes more cheerful and social, defining his understanding of sanity, similar in fact to the much earlier alienists who pursued Moral Therapy and those who ran the first asylums; the success of any treatment is identified and defined by the physician, not the patient or their relatives-this can be the patient going back to work, getting married or smiling more and being gregarious, based as it is on behaviour and acceptance of the doctor's perceptions and their treatments; the physician will write up his or her *successful efforts* whatever the thoughts or feelings of others, and usually put it down to the drugs they use, although, within reason, one drug would have been as good as another; also, did the girl have emotional reasons for being flat or at that time period experienced recreational drugs, and that was what she was hoping for when she went away with the stranger, if in fact he was a stranger or just unknown to her parents; were there any problems within the family? The physician does not ask or feel he needs to as all mental illness is formed on a disease template; did she just come awake?

In terms of perception of the treatment, this is dominated by the doctor and not the other participants. The doctor makes notes which then emerge as scientific testimony. There is no challenge to the doctor's perceptions or record. The views of the parents and daughter are not recorded but may be expressed orally so acquire no historical, thereby scientific, impact. Accordingly, drug treatment worked-accordingly.

It must be remembered that until the introduction of the monoamine hypothesis, his profession would not have been automatically agreed with by everyone. They would have been agreed with only in the asylum, where they ruled and which they controlled. The profession's expansion and its credibility as a result of the promotion of drugs and personality disorder as a wrap-around diagnosis has engendered belief by both the general public and government bodies.

Lieberman believes psychiatry has been a modern miracle, but is that simply the view of one of its practitioners imposed on *others*-patients- who cannot answer back nor largely are able to construct (due in part to the effects of the drugs Lieberman prescribes) intellectual responses. Only one group is heard, those belonging to an elite group with the greatest investment.

His narrative, meant to demonstrate his brilliant and authentic diagnostic skills, demonstrates also the appalling charlatanism of people like Reich, without perhaps acceding his own profession's similar legions of fakery.

6

In the UK NICE is the body that allocates funds on the basis of Utilitarianism, the greatest good for the greatest number at the cheapest cost. The National Health Service is costly and functions on an industrial, corporate manner, a central brand in which managers and doctors are the greatest power, with both earning far more than anyone else. NICE has tended to buy treatments that fit the equation of 'if a treatment costs 100 pounds per person and works, or appears to work for everyone, and another treatment costs 40 pounds but only works, or appears to work for 60%, then the cheaper option is preferred.' Money comes into all such calculations.

Drugs would seem a cheap option, coming with it a one drug, within reason, approach that suits industrialised or post-industrialised societies where human value is located in work and productivity. Of course drug prescriptions have probably cost the economy as those so prescribed have slowed-up cognition and their judgement is affected. Giving more considered therapies is costly. Without much intellectual content, the rationale behind psychotropic drugs is easier to grasp.

States prefer to deal with the medical profession, doctors at least, because members of ruling elites have traditionally socialised with them, may have grown up with them, doctors are a recognised power in the state alongside police authorities, and they tend to be authoritarian-personality types. Intellectually, doctors do not rock the system nor challenge accepted views.

So what is psychiatry?

Thomas Szasz[161] holds that it is '*the theory and practice of coercion*', and that is has no therapeutic intentions. It is a continuation of the 1930s and 40s tropes of control. Certainly, there is no evidence it actually works, the drugs it employs may actually be dangerous, and its high-handed methods are constantly worrying. In this I agree with Edmund Schonenberger, a lawyer who runs a collective in Zurich aimed at helping mental health patients, that the coercion routinely practised by psychiatrists infringes human rights, demonstrating that psychiatry sees itself as above the law, and represents not care but an instrument of domination.[162] Psychiatrists homing in on vulnerable patients is a blood-curdling experience for an observer let alone the victims. At such times I was reminded of the studious child, the stereotypical nerd, who has identified with his or her bullies and is in a position to eradicate his or her painful memories.

Psychiatry seems to have no plausible ideas and its ideology is self-serving. Szasz points out that there's no evidence that the psychotic wants to be cured and forcing them has caused immense suffering. Similarly, psychiatry has no real idea of what madness is and theories such as monoamine hypothesis are merely a means to camouflage their ignorance.

Edward Shorter produces the occasional downbeat estimate of psychiatry, as in *Before Prozac: The Troubled History of Mood Disorders in Psychiatry*[163] stating that the drugs do not work and there is no evidence that they do. Most contributors to the matter of Psychiatry would consider Shorter more neutral than Szasz who tends to be thought of as assuming a negative position towards his own profession. Shorter accuses Psychiatry as living in dreamland where nostology is concerned, with which I agree, pushing one unproven theory after another. The holes in DSM are enormous, more a parody of psychiatry than a science, and the monoamine hypothesis is an industry clutching at straws. Psychiatry should really have a far worse reputation than it does, but in general it is believed. That is probably the truly extraordinary part.

Nevertheless while blaming inadequate RCTs in drug testing, Shorter still believes that anecdotal estimates are valid, but as they come only from physicians I truly doubt their efficacy. There is no attempt to ascertain subjective experience of the drugs, and there must be. Physician judgement is not science although a number of psychiatrists I have spoken to believe it is.

The problem remains: psychiatry still does not understand what causes Schizophrenia even though it has supped from a number of disciplines, including genetics. No abnormalities have been identified in the brains of sufferers.[164] Yasmeen Salma confronts the very issue, or approach, of positivism in the problem of understanding human experience, suggesting that science is not the tool to understand it. A different kind of thinking is required, one not tethered

[161] Coercion as Cure: a Critical History of Psychiatry. Transaction Publishers. 2010

[162] Fundamental Criticism of Coercive Psychiatry.
https://www.academia.edu/19769384/Fundamental_criticism_of_coercive_psychiatry

[163] Oxford University Press. 2009.

[164] Yasmeen, Salma. Challenging the globalisation of biomedical psychiatry. Journal of Public Mental Health. Vol 4 issue. Pavilion Publishing (Brighton) Ltd.

simply to understanding severe mental illness as a problem that requires invasive treatment and/or intrusive practices.

If, as I believe, and my research indicates, psychotropic drugs are dangerous then how has *Asylum Psychiatry* been so successful? One answer, and the most plausible one, is that the medical profession controls and shapes reality as a result of un-conditional and un-critical respect by the general public and politicians. Their power and influence is instrumental in the passive acceptance of psychiatric views. Coercion as Szasz claims is common and seen in action (see above) it can be shocking, ideologically driven and, at times, fanatical in its convictions.

As Joanna Moncrieff points out, the media transmits the ideas of *Asylum Psychiatry*. The patient who forgets their drugs is a stock character on many TV shows, especially those about doctors, clinics and hospitals. I have never actually witnessed it. Mental illness is shown as being treated by prescriptions, drug therapy is discussed positively and only occasionally do its negative effects get reported. Other forms of therapy are occasionally mocked. Few, if any, programmes show characters wrestling with tranquilliser addiction or demonstrate the very real problems associated with the drugs. When anything of such sensitivity is transmitted, psychiatrists insist that they are wrong and patients should not be put off drug treatment.

Health Service propaganda, reviewed in *Dangers of Psychotropic Drugs*, plays a considerable part and is directly responsible for conveying an unrealistic, idealised view of psychiatry and alters in effect the reality of its efficacy. On very odd occasions the reality of psychotropic drugs is reported and argued by a physician, and these are sometimes ordinary GPs able to step outside the teaching of its own group.

When writing of psychiatry, I am reminded also of another time when another dangerous medical treatment was used ubiquitously and in this instance for thousands of years, its usage stopped only in the last century.

Bloodletting as practised by physicians was a cure-all, and throughout the time of its use physicians did not notice that it routinely killed patients. If a patient survived, it was the treatment; if a patient died then the treatment was either not applied quickly enough or thoroughly enough. Throughout the history of its use, physicians enumerated its manifold curative capacities from headaches to poisoning. I suggest that blood-taking was a major treatment for so long because it created identification of who was and who was not a genuine physician at a time when the profession faced competition from folk medicine. Only real doctors, or university doctors, could use bloodletting, as only legal physicians-registered with medical authorities- can now prescribe drugs.

Szasz suggests that psychiatry is fantasy; that is none of its applications are based on science or even actually successful. My research into the profession reveals a liminal world where truth is what its inhabitants want it to be: cures occur if they say they do: evidence is justified if they say it is. Although the medical profession, officially represented as a body, has monopolised healthcare, its achieving this is very recent and has relied on its association with the state, a group conformist and authoritarian approach, and of course the active elimination of other groups as frauds and charlatans (see *An Unusual Power: Becoming the Ruling Class*).

Doctor demographic:

According to [165] 36% of trainee doctors went to private schools indicating a well-to do background, with 56% of psychiatric trainees from minorities mainly it seems because there is less competition for these posts and their involvement may indicate prejudice. There is too little data on doctors, especially psychiatrists, where determinates of character, views, prejudices may be essential. In the UK, trainee doctors are usually from wealthy backgrounds and may therefore have limited or preferential experience of life. They may have a sense of entitlement for example. [166] A large number, in some schools as much as 80%, have parents in the professional class. Whether we appreciate it or not, each demographic group brings preconceptions to any task, and with those from entitled backgrounds a sense of superiority can be part of their cognitive toolkit. In the past when many psychiatrists were from, in the UK, the upper middle class, they would have had nothing in common with the people they treated. In other papers in *An Unknown Power* it can be seen that Alienists created their identity and power in a hierarchical relationship with the poor and dispossessed.

The final point returns to the question of physician *authoritarianism,* recalling the two aspects of this personality type. Alessandra Colaianni in A Long Shadow: Nazi doctors, moral vulnerability and contemporary medical culture, points out how many doctors became Nazi supporters, pointing out the involvement of doctors in torture and genocide over the past decades. She points to not only doctors' involvement in German concentration camps but also more recent episodes such as mercy killings after Hurricane Katrina and torture at Guantanamo Bay. She decides that situationism does not explain a pronounced authoritarian, indeed sadistic trait in doctors but can be observed as a consequence of their training. As I have noted here and elsewhere, medicine is hierarchical, with those at the very bottom-junior doctors-doing exactly what they are told by their superiors. They are not expected to speak up, nor advised to question their superiors. The hard work and frequent sleep deprivation of learning to be a doctor mean that socialisation process hastens the embedding of authoritarian behaviour patterns. She also identifies 'ambition' as part of the process of socialisation, adaptation leading to a reduction in ethical behaviour. The gruesome nature of doctoring adds to decreased sensitivity (An Unusual Power: Frankenstein, Body Snatchers and the Monster) inflicting pain and the employment of euphemisms (see DSM) to cover violent acts in research, labelling patients who ask questions (do not do as they are told) as difficult or non-compliant; detached from suffering, the suffering they cause, and thereby from reality. [167]

The other side of *authoritarianism* is believing what you are told and what you read. In this analysis, a psychiatrist who reads that a certain drug works in this particular way, is not addictive or harmful, believes it and makes no further checks: a psychiatrist who reads ECT is

165
https://www.york.ac.uk/media/che/documents/papers/researchpapers/CHERP_119_junior_doctors_training_specialities.pdf
166 https://www.theguardian.com/society/2016/jan/22/medical-school-students-wealthy-backgrounds
167
https://jme.bmj.com/content/38/7/435.long?int_source=trendmd&int_medium=trendmd&int_campaign=trendmd

fine, believes it; a psychiatrist who is told that drug-treatments deal with proven conditions initiated by monoamine hypotheses believes it. They make no checks, they do not question. If a parent, possessing authority to their minds, tells them their offspring is mad, they believe it; if it is a husband in cultures where husband have authority over their wives, they believe it. Reality is not their choice, but that of anyone who has authority.

Conclusion

I have considered a number of issues here: the doubtful nature of the monoamine hypothesis that underwrites drug treatments of mental illness-although these were started almost fifteen years before the hypothesis was published: the insufficient proof for the efficacy of drugs as a treatment for mental illness: the popularisation of drugs as products of science, not only by the medical profession but by writers in the media-magazines, newspapers, TV, with practically no focus on the possible harm of the drugs: the comparative horror commonly expressed with regards to recreational drugs, often displaying the same properties as medical drugs: the nature of the DSM and its foreshadowing in phrenology and astrology (Dr Steven Hyman, the ex-Director of US National Institute of Mental Health is recorded as dismissing it as a nightmare and out of touch with science[168], but I would go further and say it is to science what offshoots of human domesticity are to do with cleanliness): further, its descriptive terms randomly and wantonly employed to give the view of medical efficacy and control.

What stands out is the sheer lack of proof with the actual scientific context produced mainly by the association of these ideas and practices with the medical profession and its vaunted status as scientific discipline-a claim it has made for several millennium with a constant and equal unreliability. In this, individual and group authoritarianism is really the key. What equally stands out is the professions' incestuous reliance on its own ideas and proofs. The many medical papers I have researched on this matter have never-this unfortunately is not an exaggeration-cited or referenced in any way scientific arguments outside its own specialisation, thereby labelling its conclusions parochial with a narrow intellectuality that is untouched by criticism. While no man may be an island, psychiatry certainly is.

Of immense concern is the lack of oversight into psychiatric practices except by members of its own professional bodies: no one truly checks efficacy of drugs (although this is done, it is done with the same mind-set, from the viewpoint of pharmaceutical claims): no one follows up except again through psychiatric ideologies as a basis of measurement. When independents do (Joanne Moncrieff for example) they invariably arrive at different results.

---

[168] Bacopoulos-Viau, A. The Patients' Turn. Roy Porter and Psychiatry's Tales, Thirty Years On. Med. His. 2016. Vol.60 (1-18)

Monoamine hypothesis:

Certainly this can without too much effort be labelled '*the elephant in the room,*' or at least the most prominent in a very wide choice. Its scientific credentials of experimenting on animals and extrapolating the results onto human beings comes from Pavlov's famous experiments on dogs, and yet he did not then prescribe drugs to people based on his data. Challenges to Pavlov's conclusions have come from researchers who deny, rightly, a straight connection between animal experiments, human beings and human benefits. The monoamine hypothesis is not simply derisive, it is psychologically dangerous.

The Harlow and Harlow experiment[169] was set up to consider the veracity of attachment theories, the learned attachment of Pavlov and the theories of the British psychiatrist Bowlby[170] who held that attachment to the mother is innate. Harlow's experiment involved the removal of Rhesus Monkey babies from their mothers and exposing them to two wire mesh substitute mothers, one bare, the mesh showing, but with artificial milk teats and the other covered in towelling without milk teats. Operant conditioning developed by Pavlov indicated that pleasure drives focussed on sustenance would prevail and monkey babies would preference and form attachments to the bare wire mesh substitute mother providing food. In fact, the monkeys attached themselves to the wire mesh covered in towelling without sustenance provision. Maslow's hierarchy of needs, where food trounces love, was then also immediately suspect. The apparent rejection of pleasure drives as the principal motivating force should not be taken too seriously if attempting to extrapolate onto human needs as experiments did not again involve human beings but monkeys. These like the monoamine hypothesis remain hypothesis, not proven so utilising the results of any experiments on animals should not then involve unexamined practices on human beings. Remember, at no point did GPs recognise they were addicting people to tranquillisers, and now anti-depressives, as psychiatrists still refuse to believe the drugs, let alone their own authoritarian behaviour, have detrimental effects. My experience indicates they can cause personality disorder and even criminal behaviour.

---

[169] http://www.psychologyconcepts.com/harlows-studies-on-attachment/
[170] https://www.learning-theories.com/attachment-theory-bowlby.html

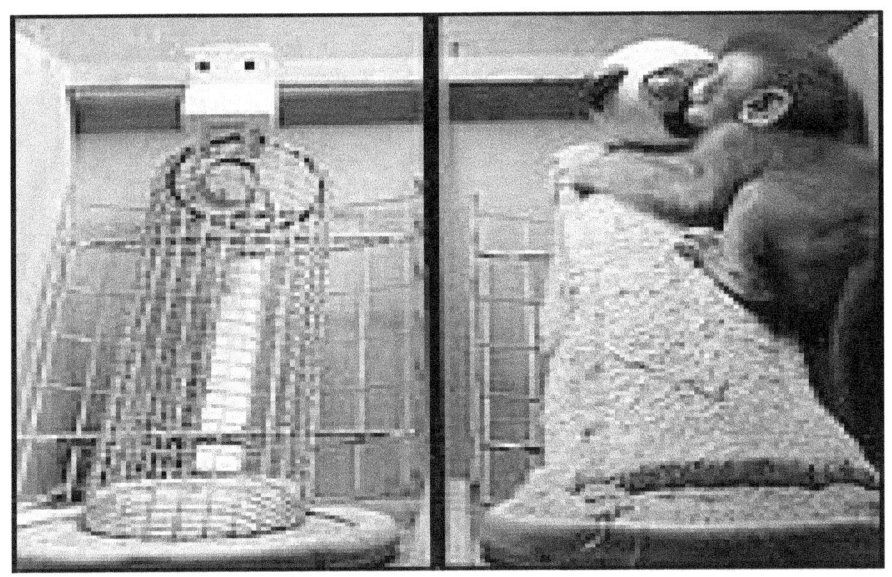

Harlow's experiment

The monoamine hypothesis came almost fifteen years after the first mood suppressant drugs were used so it does indeed look like a way of providing scientific credence to an already established practice, not a genuine advance.

This refutation of reductionism does not thereby exonerate Bowlby who believed that juvenile delinquency was caused by errant or absent mothering, the incapacity to create the prime object relation[171], and that such delinquency involved mental disorder. By doing so he related *badness* (in his view and those of his peers) with *madness*, investing personality disorder with a moral aetiology-in common with many of his profession.

Recent hypothesis:

'In most cases, depression has biological correlates but not necessarily biological causes. Emotional wounds may cause alterations in neurotransmitter levels or receptor sites. The powerful, resonant events of life may interact with brain chemistry, provoking shifts in mood

---

[171]Bretherton, Inge.THE ORIGINS OF ATTACHMENT THEORY: JOHN BOWLBY AND MARY AINSWORTH: Developmental Psychology (1992), 28, 759-775.

states, but nobody can conclusively assert where biological factors intersect with non-biological ones. The biochemical basis of depression is usually analysed from genetic and biochemical perspectives.' James Paul Pandarakalam. Certain Bio-Cognitive and Quantum Views of Depression. *American Journal of Psychiatry and Neuroscience.*

Vol. 6, No. 2, 2018, pp. 33-45. doi: 10.11648/j.ajpn.20180602.12

Dr Pandarakalam believes that cognitive therapy is viable for depression and probably other conditions not specified as schizophrenia or mania. This separation, while crucial, has been lost in the construction of mental illness as a *whole* on the basis of drug treatment for all with its corresponding leap into day to day lived existence. Drugs are prescribed if employment is lost, a parent or partner dies, a beloved cat or dog expires, if someone is tired through overwork or simply, by nature, gloomy.

Although Dr Pandaraklam's views on the nature of monoamine affects are an improvement on rationality as well as diagnosis, he misses the clear point that the results of childhood deprivation and trauma may produce pessimism, this too is a human characteristic. It is not an illness. It is not therefore likely to benefit from infusions of drugs. The range of human moods and aspects is considerable and understanding of human personalities and moods should not be shaped by false or fantasy normalities constructed by psychiatry.

DSM

This regularly produced directory/dictionary is equally worrying as very few of its assertions seems reliably scientific. It constructs stereotypes without any attempt to provide legitimate causation or proof. Its constructs, rendered as people, stand alone. These sets of cognitive habits and fixed behaviours expressed in vignettes at best, demonstrate neither positive attributes (all humans do) nor connections to others. They exist on a separate plane, without friends, family, work colleagues and hope. Are they simply products of professional fantasy, like a good portion of psychiatry appears to be?

Authoritarian:

Psychiatrists operate like an additional police force specialising in the mad: but they effectively choose who is mad. The process of diagnosis is subject to whim, and if the DSM is employed in diagnosis, *very bad science*. In the UK the diagnosis often occurs through individuals being picked up by the police and from there diagnosis as mentally ill is a certainty.

Psychiatrists, once someone is diagnosed, expect to control that person for the rest of their lives, without any concern for the psychological effect on the person or on their lives and the lives of any individuals dependent upon them. Psychiatrists are exceptionally well-paid and invariably come from elite groups, therefore have few material concerns. Their attitudes are normally constructed upon career-competition, their position within a hierarchy and financial gain, even if the latter is not a single imperative. Soliciting patients and diagnosing indiscriminately may therefore serve specific professional ends.

Psychiatrists, they rule anyone they come into contact with as a patient. My clients have also told me that they tout for custom (see above): one friend whose wife suffered from depression found himself offered outpatient treatment from the hospital his wife briefly attended and drugs from his GP. The actions of the hospital particularly irritated him as they offered his wife no genuine help, seemed confused and ill-directed and she received some help in the end from counselling. They both felt psychiatrists stereotyped people and were themselves prejudiced against the mentally ill. The GP acted as a drug pusher.

My own dealings working alongside psychiatrists, etc, convinced me that they believed they had liege rights over others: they were their patients' lords and masters and could do whatever they wanted with the people who looked to them for help: lobotomies, ECT, proscribing any drugs they desired, whatever their effects. My second conviction concerns the fact that every mental health hypothesis is form by psychiatry without reference to other ideas in other disciplines, that instead of actually checking the sincerity of such hypothesis they drug people, and do not, to make matters worse, do proper checks on the drugs' effects. As a monopoly they can: as a monopoly supported by the state, they can.

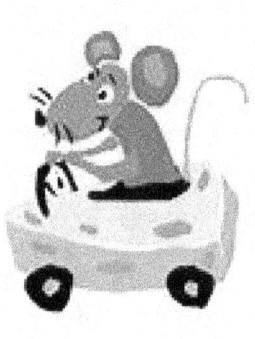

A mouse driving a car: a regular mirage seen by psychiatrists

BIBLIOGRAPHY:

Adorno, Theodor W.et al. The Authoritarian Personality: 1950: **Harper & Row.**

Bacopoulos-Viau, A. The Patients' Turn. Roy Porter and Psychiatry's Tales, Thirty Years On. Med. His. 2016. Vol.60 (1-18)

Baumeister, Alan A, et al. The Myth of Reserpine-Induced Depression: Role in the Historical Development of the Monoamine Hypothesis. Journal of the History of the Neurosciences. Basic and Clinical Perspectives. Volume 12. 2003. Issue 2.

Bennet, Charles, E/Hammond, William A, Translation. The Characters of Theophrastus A 'Translation^ with Introduction By Charles E. Bennett and William A. Hammond Professors in Cornell University Longmans, Green, and Co. 91 and 93 Fifth Avenue, New York London and Bombay 1902. http://www.archive.org/stream/charactersoftheo00theorich/charactersoftheo00theorich_djvu.txt

Berrios.G.E. Melancholia and Depression During the 19th Century: A Conceptual History. The British Journal of Psychiatry. Vol. 153. Issue 3. Sept.1988. 298.304.

Bottelier, Marco, E. The effects of Psychotropic drugs On Developing brain (ePOD) study: methods and design. BMC Psychiatry. 2014.

Bretherton, Inge.THE ORIGINS OF ATTACHMENT THEORY: JOHN BOWLBY AND MARY AINSWORTH: Developmental Psychology (1992), 28, 759-775.

Bynum, Porter, Shepherd. The Anatomy of Madness. Essays in the History of Psychiatry. Vol. 111. The Asylum and its Psychiatry. Routledge. 2004.

Davie, Niel. *"False in Doctrine and Cruel in Practice."* Henry Maudsley the M'naghten Rules and and Mental Responsibility. Unpublished paper. 2011. Universitie Lumiere Lyon. Academia edu.

Deutsch, M., & Gerard, H. B. (1955). A study of normative and informational social influences upon individual judgment. The Journal of Abnormal and Social Psychology, 51(3), 6

Digby, Anne. Madness, Morality and Medicine. A Study of the York Retreat, 1796-1914. Cambridge University Press. 1985: page 3.

Elhwuegi, Abdalla Salem. Central monoamines and their role in major depression$ Department of Pharmacology and Toxicology, Faculty of Pharmacy and Health Sciences, Ajman University of Science.

Fantie, Brown, Moger. Constant lighting conditions affect sexual behaviour and hormone levels in sexual male rats. Departments of Psychology, Physiology and Biophysics, Dalhousie University Halifax, Canada. 1984 Journals of Reproduction and Fertility Ltd.

Fernandez, Ana olea. PSYCHIATRIC DIAGNOSIS & PSYCHOTROPIC DRUGS IN LOOKED AFTER CHILDREN & YOUNG PEOPLE. Academia.edu.

Fink/Nemeroff. *The Neuroendocrine View of ECT.* Convulsive Therapy. 5 (3):296-304. 1989. Raven Press Ltd.

Foucault, Michel.
https://monoskop.org/images/1/14/Foucault_Michel_Madness_and_Civilization_A_History_of_Insanity_in_the_Age_of_Reason.pdf

Freeman, W, Watts, J. W., & Hunt, T. (Collaborator). (1942). Psychosurgery: Intelligence, emotion, and social behavior following prefrontal lobotomy for mental disorders. London, England: Baillière, Tindall & Cox.

Gray, Peter. Evolution and Human Sexuality. Yearbook of Physical Anthropology. 2013.

Griffen, Charles &Co. Textbook of Mental Diseases.. 1889.

Harkins, Stephen G. et al. The Oxford Handbook of Social Influence.

Hughes, et al. Adverse event assessment methods in published trials of psychotropic drugs: Poor reporting and neglect of emerging safety concerns. International Journal of Risk and Safety in Medicine 28 (2016) 101-1014.

Huneman, Writing the case-Pinel as Psychiatrist. Institute of Histoire et de Philosophie des Sciences et des Techniques, CNRS/Universite Paris I Sorbonne.

Jones, Colin. The Treatment of the Insane in eighteenth-and early nineteenth-century Montpelier. A Contribution to the Prehistory of the lunatic asylum in Provincial France. Medical History, 1980., 24: 371-390.

Jung, C. G. Archetypes and the Collective Unconscious (Collected Works of C.G. Jung) Princeton University Press. 1969.

Kafka, Martin P. MD. Archives of Sexual Behaviour. Vol. 26. No 4. 1997.

Kapur, S, et al. Why has it taken so long for biological psychiatry to develop clinical tests and what to do about it? Mol Psychiatry. 2012 Dec;17(12):1174-9. doi: 10.1038/mp.2012.105. Epub 2012 Aug 7.PMID:22869033

Kelman HC. Compliance, identification, and internalization: Three processes of attitude change. Journal of Conflict Resolution. 1958;2 (1) :51-60.

Kidman, Hinwood, Yeo. Journal of Neurochemistry.1976. Vol 27. Pages 293-294. Pergamon Press. Great Britain.

Klimeka, Robersona, et al: Serotonin transporter and MAO-B levels in monoamine nuclei of the human brainstem are normal in major depression. Journal of Psychiatric Research 37 (2003) 387-397.

Kraepelin,Emil
https://archive.org/stream/onehundredyearso011002mbp/onehundredyearso011002mbp_djvu.txt

MacKenzie, Charlotte. Psychiatry For the Rich, A History of Ticehurst Private Asylum, 1792-1917. Routledge, London-New York. 1992.

Mayhew, Henry. *The Longer Underworld in the Victorian Period: Authentic first person accounts by beggars, thieves and prostitutes.* 1862. Ebook by various suppliers.

Micale, Mark S/Porter, Roy. Ed. Discovering the History of Psychiatry. Oxford University Press. 1994.

Miller-Keane Encyclopedia and Dictionary of Medicine, Nursing, and Allied Health, Seventh Edition. © 2003 by Saunders

Moncrieff, Joanna, et al. The Psychoactive Effects of Psychiatric Medication: The Elephant in the Room Joanna Moncrieff M.B.B.S. , David Cohen & Sally Porter. 2013................
.... Moncrieff, Joanna. The Myth of the Chemical Cure (2007) Palgrave.

Newcombe, Russell. Psychonautics:A Model and Method for Exploring the Subjective Effects of Psychoactive drugs. #d Research Bureau. 1999.

The Treatment of the Insane in eighteenth-and early nineteenth-century Montpelier. A Contribution to the Prehistory of the lunatic asylum in Provincial France. Medical History, 1980., 24: 371-390.

Novais, Filipa, et al. *Front Psychol. 2015; 6: 1463. Published online 2015 Sep 25.*
doi: 10.3389/fpsyg.2015.01463

Pandarakalam, James Paul. Certain Bio-Cognitive and Quantum Views of Depression. *American Journal of Psychiatry and Neuroscience.*
Vol. 6, No. 2, 2018, pp. 33-45. doi: 10.11648/j.ajpn.20180602.12

Parry-Jones, William L. The Trade in Lunacy. Routledge 2013.

.............English private madhouses in the eighteenth and nineteenth centuries. Proc R Soc Med. **1973 Jul; 66(7): 659–664.**

Plante, Rebecca/Sexual Fields: Toward Sociology of Collective Sexual Life. Book Review.Ed. Adam Isaiah Green. Chicago, IL. University of Chicago, 2014.

Pliny Earle.An Examination Practice of Bloodletting for Mental Disorders.

Porter, Roy. A Social History of Madness. Stories of the Insane. Weidenfeld & Nicolson. 1987: p 167.

Read, dr. http://www.nickread.co.uk/articles/2010/03/visionary-or-disaster-a-perspective-on-william-sargant/

Richardson, J. Steven. On the of monoamine oxidase, the emotions, and adaptation to stress. International Journal of Neuroscience. May 1993. www.ncbi.nlm.nih.gov/pubmed/8083027
Savanna, Stephane. Can Rats Reason? Psychology of Consciousness: Theory, Research and Practice. 2015. Vol 2. No 4. 404-429.

Schonenberger, Edmund. Fundamental Criticism of Coercive Psychiatry. *BMJ* 2017;357:j2904. Pub. 13 July 2017.

Scull, Mackenzie, Hervey: Masters of Bedlam: The Transformation of the Mad-Doctors' Trade. Princeton University Press. 1996.

Sparks, A, et al. PSYCHIATRIC DRUGS AND COMMON FACTORS: AN EVALUATION OF RISKS AND BENEFITS FOR CLINICAL PRACTICE. Psychiatric Drugs and Common Factors.

Shorter, Edward. History of Psychiatry: From the Era of the Asylum to the Age of Prozac. Wiley, 1997.
..................Before Prozac: The Troubled History of Mood Disorders in Psychiatry. Oxford University Press. 2009.

Mrs. Sushma. C1*, et al. The International Journal of Indian Psychology ISSN 2348-5396 (e) | ISSN: 2349-3429 (p) Volume 3, Issue 2, No.8, DIP: 18.01.153/20160302 ISBN: 978-1-329-95395-6 http://www.ijip.in | January - March, 2016

Szasz, Thomas Dr. Coercion as Cure: a Critical History of Psychiatry. Transaction Publishers. 2010

Tyrer, Casey, Ferguson Personality Disorder in Perspective.. The British Journal of Psychiatry. 1991.

Weiner, et al. American Psychiatric Association. Committee on Electroconvulsive Therapy. The practice of electroconvulsive therapy: recommendations for treatment, training and privileging. Washington DC. American Psychiatric Publishing. 2001.

Wilkin, S. An Unusual Power: Madhouses: Sane or insane?https://www.researchgate.net/publication/320173717_An_Unusual_Power_Madhouses_Sane_or_Insane

Wilson, Sylia, et al. US National Library of Medicine. National Institute of Health.

Yasmeen, Salma. Challenging the globalisation of biomedical psychiatry. Journal of Public Mental Health.Vol 4 issue. Pavilion Publishing (Brighton) Ltd.

Yoganathan, N. /Dr J Willis. The Madness of Psychiatry (in 21st Century UK): Large Group Analytic Perspective. Academia.edu